Eating at school - Making healthy choices

Report of the European Forum
Strasbourg, 20-21 November 2003

organised jointly by the Council of Europe and
the World Health Organization, Regional Office for Europe

Rapporteur: Ian Young, NHS Health Scotland
WHO, Regional Office for Europe

French edition:
L'alimentation à l'école – faire le choix de la santé
ISBN 92-871-5573-9

Cover design: Morten Strunge Meyer, thanks to The Danish Veterinary and Food Administration
Layout: Pre-press unit, Council of Europe
Council of Europe Publishing
F-67075 Strasbourg Cedex

ISBN 92-871-5574-7
©Council of Europe, February 2005
Printed in Germany

Contents

Preface 7

Introduction 9

Hors-d'œuvre 11

Opening addresses 13

Chairman's introduction
Bent Egberg Mikkelsen, Danish Veterinary and Food Administration 13

Welcome address
Peter Baum, Council of Europe 19

Young Minds 2002-2003 – forward ever, backward never
Sarah Hunter and Tara Mcardle 23

Introductory overview – Health behaviour and nutrition among
school-aged children
Lea Maes, Ghent University 29

Keynote address – Eating at school – A European Study
*Fannie de Boer, Wageningen University and Reseach Centre,
the Netherlands* 35

Participants' interviews
Ian Young, rapporteur 45

Young Minds forum workshop 51

I – Healthy eating in schools
Facilitator: Jeltje Snel 59

Is there a healthy school meal?
Ines Heindl, University of Flensburg, Germany 59

Hungry for success: A whole approach to school meals in Scotland
Gillian Kynoch, Scottish Executive Health Department 67

How can school influence children's food choice and improve their diet?
Isabelle Loureiro, Escola Nacional de Salude Publica, Portugal 77

Discussion 85

II - How to provide healthy food in schools
Facilitator: Vivian Rasmussen 87

Healthy eating in the traditional school meals system. The role of the private food operator
Richard Coudyser, Sodexho Education, France 87

How to provide healthy food in schools: School fruit programmes as a short cut to promoting healthy eating in schools – The Norwegian experience
Anniken Owren Aarum, Directorate for Health and Social Affairs, Norway ... 95

The home-made lunchbox – Has it got a future?
Doris Kuhness, Styria Vitalis Organisation, Austria 99

Discussion 101

III – Whole school approach
Facilitator: Maria Vaz de Almeida 103

School food policy: linking with The Netherlands healthy schools action programme
Goof Buijs, National Institute of Health Promotion and Disease Prevention, the Netherlands 103

Promoting good personal health care and healthy consumption habits through a good school climate
Jean-Claude Vuille, Department of Public Health, Switzerland 109

Health and education – Intersectoral role of school nutrition and nutrition education
Irena Simcic, Institute of Education, and Cirila Hlastan Ribic, Ministry of Health, Republic of Slovenia 113

Discussion 117

IV – Partnerships for healthy choices
Facilitator: Cristine Deliens 119

We decide what we eat: Active involvement of students in developing school meal policies
Bjarne Bruun Jensen, University of Education, Denmark 119

Eating at school: The school and parents as partners – Utopia or reality?
Patricia Melotte and Christophe Content, Association des parents de l'Ecole communale Clair Vivre, Belgium 131

Contents

National inter-agency co-operation regarding nutrition in schools
Michel Chauliac, Ministère de la Santé, France 137

Discussion 151

Poster papers

Policy reviews (posters 4, 5, 12, 13 and 22) 153

Partnerships (posters 1, 9, 11, 15, 18 and 23) 156

Education and training (posters 2, 3, 6, 7, 16, 21) 161

Utilising research (posters 10, 14 and 21) 165

Changing traditions (posters 24 and 25) 168

The environment and sustainability (posters 17, 18 and 25) 170

Closing remarks
Bent Egberg Mikkelsen 175

Rapporteur's reflections
Ian Young 177

Appendix 1: List of participants 181

Appendix 2: Poster papers 195

Appendix 3: Some useful websites 199

The Council of Europe

The Council of Europe is a political organisation, which was founded on 5 May 1949 by ten European countries in order to promote greater unity between its members. It now numbers 46 member states.

The main aims of the organisation are to promote democracy, human rights and the rule of law, and to develop common responses to political, social, cultural and legal challenges in its member states. Since 1989 it has integrated most of the countries of central and eastern Europe and supported them in their efforts to implement and consolidate their political, legal and administrative reforms.

Its permanent headquarters are in Strasbourg (France) and by Statute it has two constituent organs: the Committee of Ministers, composed of the Ministers of Foreign Affairs of the 46 member states, and the Parliamentary Assembly, comprising delegations from the 46 national parliaments. The Congress of Local and Regional Authorities of Europe represents the entities of local and regional self-government within the member states.

The European Court of Human Rights is the judicial body competent to adjudicate complaints brought against a state by individuals, associations or other contracting states on grounds of violation of the European Convention on Human Rights.

Partial Agreement in the social and public health field

Where a lesser number of member states of the Council of Europe wish to engage in some action in which not all their European partners desire to join, they can conclude a "Partial Agreement" which is binding on themselves alone.

The Partial Agreement in the social and public health field was concluded on this basis in 1959. At present, the Partial Agreement in the social and public health field has 18 member states.[1]

The principal areas of activity include:

- protection of public health and especially the health of the consumer
- rehabilitation and integration of people with disabilities.

---

1.   Austria, Belgium, Cyprus, Denmark, Finland, France, Germany, Ireland, Italy, Luxembourg, The Netherlands, Norway, Portugal, Slovenia, Spain, Sweden, Switzerland, United Kingdom of Great Britain and Northern Ireland.

The activities are entrusted to committees of experts, which are responsible to a steering committee for each area.

The work of these Partial Agreement committees occasionally results in the elaboration of conventions or agreements, but the more usual outcome is the drawing-up of recommendations to member states in the form of resolutions adopted by the Committee of Ministers. The resolutions should be considered as statements of policy for national policy makers. Governments have actively participated in their formulation: the delegates on the Partial Agreement committees are both experts in the field in question and responsible for the implementation of government policy in their national ministries.

A less formal procedure is the publication of general guidelines intended to serve as a model for member states. Each government can interpret these guidelines in accordance with its own law and practice in the matter.

Furthermore, scientific reports aimed at informing both governments and experts in the field are published on specific questions of current concern.

Nutrition, food safety and consumer health

While European policy regarding food safety has until recently been based on the concept of monitoring food quality in microbiological and chemical terms, it has been clear from certain dietary habits that a more positive approach to nutrition is needed and that diet should be stressed as a primary health factor. Therefore in 1998 a Committee of experts on nutrition, food safety and consumer health was set up, one of whose tasks is to organise fora for the discussion of various aspects of nutrition in Europe. The results of the fora are translated into resolutions and/or guidelines.

It is within this context that the present report has been prepared.

Aims of the forum "Eating at school – making healthy choices"

The Council of Europe, jointly with the World Health Organization, Regional Office for Europe, organised this forum to:

- Promote healthy eating in schools as an integral part of healthy lifestyles:
- Foster co-operation to enable children to eat healthy meals in a pleasant environment in their schools;
- Review different European approaches to the provision of food in schools;
- Make proposals for follow-up activities to be pursued by the Council of Europe.

The Forum was held in Strasbourg, France on 20 and 21 November 2003 and was attended by 143 participants from 27 countries. An emerging view from the forum was that the issues are so important that a resolution and guidelines should be drafted for consideration by the Council of Europe. This is an important follow-up activity to the forum.

A task force played a central role in planning the forum and a wider ad hoc group played a supportive part in the planning for the event. The membership of these groups is given in Appendix I.

Acknowledgements

Special thanks are extended to the following

- The Ad hoc group on nutrition in schools and its chairman, Bent Mikkelsen.
- Fanny De Boer, who conducted the European Survey commissioned by the Netherlands Nutrition Centre, the main results of which were presented at the forum.
- The Young Minds group for their active participation and valuable contribution.

Appetisers served at the forum .....
What some delegates had to say.....

"As a *school principal, I think it is important to link the issues of school quality with the health promoting school and nutrition/food provision. They are not separate issues.*"
Bauke Houtsma, The Netherlands.

"*After the conference (at Egmond) we decided to institute healthy options in our school. We replaced sweets with fruit bars and fresh fruit salads.*"
Tara McArdle, Young Minds.

"*School catering is at the crossroads*"
Richard Coudyser, France.

"*The World Health Organization is promoting fruit and vegetables in a new joint initiative with The Food and Agriculture Organisation. This is the food and nutrition action plan - governments will be assessed on what they are doing.*"
Aileen Robertson, WHO.

"*School Nutrition Action Groups (SNAGS) played an important role in sharing a common disappointment about school meals and shared a vision about where they (school meals) might go.*"
Gillian Kynoch, Scotland.

"*We have this idea that we want cheaper and cheaper food, but good food costs and we need to learn this.*"
Aileen Robertson, WHO.

"*It costs around 10 million Euros annually.*" (The Norwegian subsidy for fruit in schools)
Anniken Owren Aarum, Norway.

"*We need to give young people practical support so that they have the knowledge and skills to cope when they live independently.*"
Jennifer Woolfe, England.

"70% to 80% of the food eaten in the EU today is processed, therefore understanding connections with the land is only one issue, pupils need to know about the realities of food processing too".
Michel Clevenot, France.

"It has become evident that the crisis of the health system is an unrecognised crisis of the education system".
Ines Heindl, Germany.

" The school is a good starting point but coherence is important."
Bent Egberg Mikkelsen, Chairman.

"What is a good school climate? An operational response would be: do people feel well? Are there low levels of bullying in the school? Are there good relationships between pupils and teachers in the school? As to how create a good school climate: if the health promoting school activities are integrated into general school development it seems to be important. Also schools need to set their own agenda and priorities."
Jean-Claude Vuille, Switzerland.

"From these experiences it is clear the words and concepts we use are crucial for the way health is viewed in school practice. Instead of nutrition projects, it is perhaps more recommendable to deal with projects about 'food, culture and the environment' – if we want to collaborate with young people and to involve them in the dialogue as genuine participants".
Bjarne Bruun Jensen, Denmark.

"In our study in Sweden the crowded dining rooms had the most scrap waste."
Mette Kjörstad, Sweden

"Coming together is a beginning, keeping together is progress, working together is success."
Henry Ford, Ford Motor Corporation.
Mr Ford did not actually attend the forum but his spirit was evoked in poster 23 from The Netherlands!

Please read on and find out not only who did attend the forum, but what they had to say about the issues and what the Task Force set up by the Council of Europe plans to do about it.

Eating at school – Making healthy choices

Bent Mikkelsen, Danish Veterinary and Food Administration

*The opening address at the forum was given by its chairman **Bent Mikkelsen** of The Nutrition Division of the Danish Veterinary and Food Administration. The following are the highlights of his presentation.*

There is an increasing focus on children's nutrition and health and in this respect school plays an important role. Thus, I am delighted that the Council of Europe has initiated work by experts designed to contribute to promoting healthier food in European schools. On behalf of the task force which has planned this forum, I am also very pleased to be able to bid so many participants a warm welcome to this forum which I hope will make an active contribution to the Council's work in this area. In particular, I am extremely satisfied that so many European countries are represented and, thanks to the support of the French Government, that it has been possible to welcome delegations from a number of central and eastern European countries.

I am very happy that the work of the Council of Europe's ad hoc group can take as its starting point the significant project which the European Network of Health Promoting Schools (ENHPS) has carried out, and continues to carry out, on school health promotion. Nutrition, of course, is closely related to other health-promoting activities taking place in schools and in this context we are fortunate to be able to draw on the experiences from the ENHPS co-operation with the Young Minds network.

This is important because the objective of healthy food at schools cannot be achieved by theorists and health professionals alone sitting behind their desks. If the initiatives are to have an effect, they must be based on a collaboration with those who will put healthier ways of living into practice on a daily basis, not least the young people themselves. Thus, we also extend a welcome to Young Minds and their active participation in this forum.

Background

There are serious reasons for holding a forum such as this. The development in the eating habits of young people and nutrition-related diseases is alarming. Globally, the incidence of obesity has risen over the past 30-40 years, and the same applies to the incidence of associated diseases, for example diabetes type

2. WHO has identified the obesity epidemic as one of the biggest threats to human health and worldwide there are now more people who are overweight than underweight (WHO, 2000).

If obesity continues to increase at the same rate, up to 40 % of all Europeans will suffer from obesity by the year 2030 (IOTF/WHO, 2002). It is particularly the increasing incidence of overweight and obesity among children and young people which is so worrying. In Denmark, there has been a threefold increase over the past 25 years (Danish Nutrition Council 2002). However, it is still worth noting that even though the principal problem here is excessive food consumption and an incorrect mix of foods combined with inadequate physical activity, insufficient food supplies are also a problem in some countries, in particular for socially vulnerable groups.

One of the areas which has received attention with regard to preventative strategies against obesity and overweight concerns the efforts being made in schools – here diet and nutrition at schools can constitute an important element.

Four important themes

As pointed out by Young (2002), food at schools is a complex phenomenon which does not just cover the food which is provided, but also the other activities connected to food including how diet and nutrition are included in the teaching. The planning task force has tried to ensure that this complexity is reflected in the forum's four sessions:

1. Firstly, it is necessary to draw up an outline of health behaviour and nutrition among school-age children and then present the main results from the European survey, which has been started on the initiative of the Council of Europe. This is explored in the opening session.

In the first session, we focus on the different nutritional and health aspects of eating in school. For example, must a fibre-rich diet be followed to a greater extent with more fruit and vegetables being consumed, combined with a reduced consumption of high fat, high-energy products? Must the intake of sugar in the form of soft drinks be limited, and if so, how? Is there a need for dietary standards at schools and what form can we envisage these taking?

2. The second session will attempt to answer the following question: how to provide healthy food in schools? Despite the fact that school life varies enormously from country to country, there is one aspect in common. Namely the fact that one cannot spend a long day at school without a proper lunch. However, the ways of meeting this need are, on the other hand, extremely varied. This applies just as much to the

various eating habits as to the practical framework governing the consumption of food. The different practical arrangements range from schemes where the food is simply based on lunch boxes brought from home to those where snacks, finger foods and wraps are sold from tuck shops to well-established schemes where the food is centrally prepared and served in dedicated canteens. There is also a difference in whether the food constitutes a main meal or a morning snack or a between-meal snack just as there are numerous different traditions applying to the financial subsidies given to the various schemes. In some countries school food is free while in other countries the pupils pay part or the entire cost of the food.

3. In the third session we will look at how schools can try to integrate food served at school with teaching in nutrition and healthy dietary habits and an increased focus on physical activity at school. This will happen under the title "whole school approach". It is especially important to emphasise the significance of physical activity. One-sided efforts to benefit healthy food schemes and eating habits will only have a weak effect if they are not combined with more physical activity. The necessity of physical activity in combination with healthy nutrition is well documented (Mathiesen et al. 2003). Thus, it is important not to consider school food in isolation but to look at it as an integrated part of the other health-promoting efforts being implemented at schools. Here, it is worthwhile drawing attention to the initiative, which the ENHPS network for health-promoting schools has taken in this area (Young, ENHPS, 2002).

4. In the fourth and final session, we will focus on the question 'What action can be taken?' Promoting healthy eating habits involves both individual and social strategies. Here, there are roles for the public authorities at all levels, the health system, private organisations and industry. The concept of partnerships plays an important role in this respect. For none of the individual players can meet the huge challenge of working for healthier school food. Non-governmental organisations and businesses are also important. I am very happy to see so many NGOs represented on the list of participants, and in particular that there are a number of catering enterprises at this forum which are actively supporting the idea of healthy food at schools in the form of presentations and sponsorships. The responsibility towards health, which food enterprises have with regard to nutrition, has received considerable focus within the past six months. Within the environmental area, we have for several years been seeing visionary companies taking the lead in promoting an environmental approach in their products and production, and we can now see signs that health concerns are spreading. In the USA, we have seen shareholders of food companies starting to demand that these companies take their responsibilities towards health seriously. I am convinced that partnerships with key players will be decisive for progress in this area.

It is important to emphasise that discussion and debate about the multifaceted subject of school food is important within this forum. Thus, time has been allocated for discussion as part of each session. It is our hope that participants will take an active part in these talks and that it will be possible to debate some of the expert statements as well as the more controversial topics. For example, are school food and institutionalised meals the only correct solution to the issue of providing food at schools? And who after all should pay? Where does the boundary lie between parental responsibility and that of the schools and society at large? And can the food companies make a positive contribution in this area? Questions such as these are necessary to discuss if we want to be able to lay down a future strategy for healthy food in schools.

What comes next? This forum is, of course, not a conclusion to the initiative which the Council of Europe has taken. The significant data about the subject which are being presented, and all the good ideas, visions and proposals that are made will be included in this report. The task force will follow this up and discuss turning the recommendations into action.

It is also important that nutritional researchers take up the challenge concerning the need for research, which will be identified, and that it takes place in a European collaboration. It is worth noting that a number of researchers are gathering after this forum to discuss the possibilities of being able to test some of the research challenges in concrete projects.

References

Richelsen, B. et al. (2002). *The Danish Obesity Epidemic.* Danish Nutrition Council.

Husby, Ida (2000). *Mad og måltider. En fælles investering i sundhed og trivsel.* Danish National Board of Health (Sundhedsstyrelsen).

IOTF/WHO (2002). *Obesity in Europe – the case for action.* The International Obesity
Task Force – European Association for the Study of Obesity. 2002.

Mathiesen, J. et al (2003). *Diet and physical activity* [in Danish] Food report, Danish Food Administration 2003:03.

Young, I. (2002). *Conference report- Education & Health in partnership – European conference on linking education with health promotion in schools.* NIGZ/WHO 2002.

Young, I. (2002). *Is healthy eating all about nutrition?* BNF Nutrition bulletin vol. 27, 7-12.

WHO (2000). *Obesity: preventing and managing the global epidemic.* Report of a WHO consultation on obesity. WHO Technical Report Series, no. 840, 2000.

Welcome address

Peter Baum, Directorate General III for Social Cohesion, Council of Europe

May I welcome you to the Council of Europe on behalf of the Secretary General. It is a great pleasure for me to see you here today.

I first wish to describe the institutional context in which this forum on school meals is taking place, and then to set it against the more general background of our programme of activities in the sphere of public health and consumer protection. With its 46 member states, representing a population of over 800 million, the Council of Europe is truly a pan-European intergovernmental organisation, which fulfils the following roles:

- safeguarding human rights, pluralist democracy and the rule of law;
- strengthening democratic stability in Europe;
- enhancing knowledge of Europe's cultural identity and cultural diversity and fostering their development;
- reinforcing social cohesion and social justice;
- seeking solutions to the problems faced by European society, through a whole range of activities.

These are the objectives pursued by the Committee of Ministers, the organisation's highest decision-making body, through the programme of activities implemented under its supervision.

The same objectives are shared by other Council of Europe bodies: the Parliamentary Assembly, the European Court of Human Rights and the Congress of Local and Regional Authorities of the Council of Europe.

By granting consultative status to over 350 non-governmental organisations, the Council of Europe has also established a genuine partnership with the citizens of Europe.

DG III, the Directorate General for Social Cohesion, seeks solutions to problems arising in the social, health and public health fields. In social policy matters our strategy is to focus on combating poverty and social exclusion in a number of areas: housing, education and training, employment, income distribution and the social services.

The Council of Europe also establishes Partial Agreements, an adaptable form of co-operation enabling a group of states to engage in activities of interest to them.

It is one of those Partial Agreements, the Partial Agreement in the Social and Public Health Field, with 18 member states and eight observer states, which is active in the sectors of public health and rehabilitation and integration of people with disabilities. This major forum is being organised by the Division of that Partial Agreement.

However, would it not be more advantageous if all 46 member states of the Council of Europe could benefit from the excellent work done under this Partial Agreement and the results achieved?

The answer is implicit in the question. The will indeed exists to extend the Partial Agreement's sectors of activity to all Council of Europe member states.

We considered it a tangible step in that direction to invite all 46 member states to participate in this forum. I am particularly pleased that many countries have accepted our invitation and are represented at the forum today. This is a very encouraging sign.

More specifically, our work programme in the public health field covers the following:

- nutrition and food safety;
- materials coming into contact with food;
- flavouring substances;
- pharmaceutical products;
- and cosmetic products.

The Committee of Experts on Nutrition, Food Safety and Consumer Health, which is made up of experts appointed by the national authorities, draws up resolutions, guidelines, scientific reports and other instruments. Its programme covers sectors as varied as nutrition in hospitals, functional foods, food supplements, high-energy drinks, stored product protection and, of course, nutrition in schools.

One of the committee's key tasks is organising European fora, bringing together people from different backgrounds to debate and exchange information on topical issues. The Committee of Experts set up a working group, chaired by Dr Mikkelsen, who is also chairing the forum, with the very task of organising this two-day event.

I wish to take this opportunity to thank Dr Mikkelsen and the members of the working group, as well as my colleagues, Laurent Lintermans, Sheila Boulajoun,

Audrey Malaisé and Lindsay Chestnutt, for all their hard work in preparing the forum.

However, we could not have held this event without you. I welcome the fact that so many of you accepted our invitation to come and discuss the subject of school meals and propose improvements to the current approach and I thank you wholeheartedly for being here.

It has become almost traditional to hold a forum on a specific nutrition-related subject every two or three years. The papers presented at this forum and the discussions and conclusions will subsequently be studied by a group of experts responsible for devising measures to be implemented by the member states in the field concerned.

Our theme this year is hence our children's eating habits and health. This is a matter of concern for us all and represents a huge challenge. How could we fail to be moved by the significant increase in the number of children who do not eat a balanced diet, the most visible sign of which is the growing number of children all over Europe who are obese? How could we disregard this trend, which not only affects the well-being of children - and of the future adults active in tomorrow's society - but also raises significant concerns as to the long-term health implications and the cost to society? One response to this complex situation lies in education and learning, which is, I believe, often a source of solutions. The earlier children are made aware of healthy eating habits and are offered easy ways of adopting them, the lower the risk that they will develop health problems due to a bad diet. Schools and all the professionals contributing to schoolchildren's well-being - that is to say all of you here today - have an essential role to play. Your presence at this forum shows you have understood this.

I hope that, as was the case with the forum on nutrition in hospitals, your conclusions will serve as a basis for recommendations on healthy eating in school, suitable for adoption by the Committee of Ministers. I also hope that, when you return to your home countries, you will pass on the ideas raised at the forum to your colleagues and that the network of experts involved in the Council's work in this field will continue to monitor the situation in the member states, so as to ensure that real progress is made regarding the food served in schools.

I wish you every success in your work and thank you for your attention.

Young Minds 2002-2003
Forward ever, backward never

Sarah HUNTER and Tara McARDLE, pupils at Plockton High School, Scotland.

The issues of student participation and international collaboration are explored in this presentation by two high school pupils who are fully involved in Young Minds. To find out more about Young Minds read on, and also refer to the forum workshop.

My name is Sara Hunter, I am 15 years old, and I am a pupil at Plockton High School in the West Highlands of Scotland. I am attending this Conference today as a member of the Young Minds group of my school, along with my fellow pupil Tara McArdle, whom I will introduce to you shortly. Both of us have been members of the Young Minds project for one and half years, since March 2002.

I should like to give you a little of the background to our involvement in the Young Minds project which ran from March and culminated in the conference at Egmond aan Zee, in Holland, at the end of September 2002. Between 15 and 20 schools from Europe took part. The project was divided into three broad sections. Firstly, Food and Nutrition in schools – what can pupils do to improve the quality of meals, snacks and drinks on sale at break-times? Secondly, Drugs and Alcohol – what can pupils do to stem the tide of these dangers to themselves and their fellow pupils? Thirdly, Well-being in schools – what can we do to improve the environment of the school to make it a more positive and welcoming one for young people? Plockton High School was teamed up with schools in the Czech Republic, Denmark and the Netherlands to look at ways of improving nutrition in schools, and to come up with practical and effective ways for so doing. It was not enough just to have the vision: it was all important to realise it, to make it happen.

It is crucial to the success of any project that the people affected by it should have ownership of it. In a school, that simply means that if the pupils take the initiative and share it with their fellow pupils and staff, then there is every chance of success.

The Young Minds project is designed to raise awareness in teenagers and pre-teenagers about the importance of healthy eating. It also aims to change and improve the food on offer, as well as attitudes towards food in school. So Young Minds for us is part of the continuing health alarms going off all over the western world at the present time. The project is one step towards ensuring that the next generation leads a long and full life, free of disease.

Of course, there are many questions to be answered. What is wholesome food? Is it a tasty or a boring phenomenon? Do we exclude all that is not wholesome? Or is it true that a little of what you fancy does you good? Can we only go so far, and hope that we can persuade young people to include some healthy options in their diet? How do we, in fact, change attitudes? Can we hope to overturn an entire eating culture?

After all, Scotland is the home of the deep-fried chocolate bar, and has one of the highest rates of heart disease in western Europe, although the good news is that these rates are coming down. Well, we Young Minders set about our project in Plockton High School by trying to find out some answers. Our research was done through questionnaires, surveys and direct communication with pupils. We wanted to find out specifically the following things. One, was the choice of poor food due simply to pupils being uneducated on nutritional needs? And by poor food, we meant fatty and sugary options, without a reasonable balance of essential nutrients. Or was it the case that the school was just not providing healthy options? Or was it a more complicated issue – did young people see healthy eating simply as 'uncool', and unnecessary interference from adults? Or was it that young people were mostly from family backgrounds that saw eating healthily as far too expensive an option? Or did people believe that if food was enjoyable, then it was good for you, therefore burgers, chips and deep-fried chocolate were as healthy as anything else?

The results were surprising. Most pupils were quite clear about the need for a balanced diet, and knew about protein, complex carbohydrates, vitamins, and minerals. They also knew that an exclusive diet of chips and burgers was not good for them. And most said they would go for healthier options if they were made available.

Our enquiries showed that many pupils did not have breakfast in the morning before coming to school, and that many could not concentrate properly in their classes during lessons before lunch. They often responded to hunger by hastily eating a chocolate bar in the short break and that was all. After intense discussion within our group, we decided that this was an issue that we should tackle, and we decided that the school should provide wholesome breakfast choices at low or at least reasonable cost. Thus the Breakfast Club was born. My fellow pupil Tara will go into the effects of this in detail in a moment. But the point was that the vision had begun to happen.

Our studies also showed, as indicated, that many young people did wish for a healthier range of options at school, but felt the school, or the commercial company supplying the school, provided far too wide a selection of crisps and sweets. This encouraged a lot of children, especially the younger ones, to fill up on chocolate at lunchtimes instead of having a proper meal.

We took a good look at this problem, and worked in various ways with our Danish, Czech and Dutch partners, on the Young Minds website and on-line sharing ideas about what made for healthy eating, how we changed attitudes, what guidance we as young people could give our own contemporaries, how we could punch home our message. We designed food pyramids which enabled us to share common solutions about communicating and reinforcing healthy eating and we were 'on a roll'.

My fellow pupil, Tara did not attend the Egmond aan Zee conference last year, but remained in Scotland as a member of the home team. During the conference we chatted on-line with the home team and asked them to come up with ideas concerning nutrition. Tara was an active contributor, and as this year both she and I are studying Home Economics, I'm very glad she now has her chance to attend a conference on Food and Nutrition.

Hello, my name is Tara McArdle, I am 16 years old, and I am delighted to continue this report.

Well, did we keep rolling? We decided two things after September 2002. One was to keep asking our friends and fellows at school what they wanted as improvements in their food choices; the other was to push hard and make desirable changes. The title of this presentation is 'Forward Ever, Backward Never', and we worked hard in that spirit to alter the attitudes, and diets of our school in favour of a wholesome eating culture. We found Young Minds to be most effective when the ideas thought up and carried out were those of the pupils themselves because this meant the pupils were deciding how they wanted the problem solved, so that when change came they were happy to go along with it. This made for a lot of successful positive developments.

First of all we looked at the school tuck shop. This is a little shop where traditionally soft drinks and chocolate bars, crisps and sweets are on sale. It is a typically British institution. At one point, the tuck shop was managed by the school, but now it is run by an outside company, which controls the school canteen. With the help of the staff and the agreement of the company, we changed the culture overnight. We got rid of the traditional sugar-laden chocolate bars and introduced healthier fruit bars with reduced fat content. We removed fizzy drinks and introduced both still and sparkling water, and healthy fruit drinks. Additionally, we introduced snacks such as plain biscuits and cheese, and fruit salad, both of which are now very popular. And we added to that vegetable pasta and tuna snacks, along with fresh fruit. And I am glad to say that water is very popular as well. It seems to be the new discovery. Lots of boys and girls were consuming sweet, fizzy drinks after sports in order to quench their thirst. Now they go for water or fruit juice. Some members of staff say they notice an improvement in the behaviour and concentration of such pupils when they come to their classes after sports. Certainly, it seems to me that in a centrally heated school, providing water seems be common sense. It is so easy to become dehydrated.

But we did not stop there. As the tuck shop opens only during breaks, we decided it would be a good idea to install water fountains around the school, as pupils were saying they were often thirsty at change-over of classes. It was a popular move, and I am glad to say that some of the more juvenile pupils have now stopped using them to spray water over their friends as they pass. I have to say that I think we were helped by images in the press showing sports stars and celebrities encouraging young people to drink more water.

Secondly, we looked at attitudes. We found that lots of young people were glad of the changes they themselves had suggested and introduced, because the new approach had upgraded their lives and made them look better and feel better. But some people viewed healthy eating and proper healthy lunches as 'uncool', and they would not be seen dead being anything but 'cool', so we hit upon the idea of providing a vending machine selling healthy snacks, sandwiches, water and fruit juice. Vending machines are definitely 'cool', and even some of those who choose chips, or pizza will use them without losing their 'street cred'. We Young Minders think that tackling the whole business of attitudes is the real key to changing eating habits. To help change attitudes still further, we began a poster campaign to promote the whole concept of healthy eating, and encourage people to choose the healthy option. These posters encourage them to think about food and educate them to decide what the healthy option is. We need to work closely with our partner schools on the attitude question, because if we get answers to that, we've won half the battle.

Thirdly, we had a good think about the menus the school canteen was offering at lunchtime.

The school canteen offers plenty of pizza, chips, burgers, along with cooked vegetables, and there is no denying that pupils like this diet because they like the taste and the texture of the stuff. They are used to it, and it gives them plenty of energy. The problem with it is that it is unvaried in its content from day to day. It is very fatty and heavy. We have succeeded in getting the canteen to introduce a healthy food bar, featuring tuna fish, cottage cheese, and egg with many green and red vegetables and fruit, dressed in low-fat yoghurt. This is beginning to prove popular but we still have a lot of work to do on the main food-bar, especially as regards the fatty content. I believe this will come with time. Of course we all need some fat, some sugar, some chocolate – after all, a little of what you fancy does you good. But not a lot! We have already succeeded in introducing a chip-free day. What is really encouraging is that the fizzy drinks and the traditional chocolate bars have gone, and there is now bottled water on sale, and plenty of fruit salad. We shall keep working on this, and I believe we shall be helped by the Regional Authority and the Scottish Government, which is concerned about the bad eating habits of Scottish schoolchildren, levels of obesity, and poor school performance. We intend to ask our fellow pupils by means of questionnaires not just what they would like to see on the menu at lunchtime but how they would like to change the environment itself to make it 'cool'. We would like to offer a list of possible meals that have a good nutritional content but do not include chips, burgers, and pizza. We do not wish to exclude these foods: we want to improve them nutritionally, but also expand the list of options. This is where we look forward to working at the conference with our partner schools to look together at menus, and to look at ways of altering perceptions.

Lastly, I return to the Breakfast Club where the revolution really began. This is still an important and integral part of our school day. Our fellow pupils have told us they come to school not having had breakfast for different reasons. We all come to school from fair distances, and bus journeys last from twenty minutes to forty-five minutes. Some pupils cannot eat very early in the morning, and feel hungry only when they arrive at school. Others have no one to prepare breakfast for them. Others have no time to take breakfast. Yet others are hungry even after having breakfast. The Breakfast Club enables all of them to kick-start their brains for a day's learning, and provides them with the means to concentrate on their lessons. The menu includes reduced fat and sugar cereal, including an oats-based porridge on Fridays, breakfast bars, bacon, fruit juice, milk and toast, and the prices are very reasonable. We shall not give that up, nor any of the other changes we have rolled out in realising our vision, because the benefits of the Breakfast Club should be the benefits of any other meal or snack taken during the school day.

But we are not complacent, and this is where the Young Minds projects are crucial: we must continue to move forward by exchanging views and ideas with other countries – that way we can learn what we have in common and also what is new and what we should be trying out at home. That is why Sara and I are so happy to be here, and looking forward to playing our full part in the events of the conference.

Health behaviour and nutrition among school-aged children

Lea MAES, professor of Health Promotion and Medical Sociology, Ghent University, Belgium

The following are highlights from the presentation, which provided a health behaviour research context for the work of the forum.

In the 2001/2 survey of the Health Behaviour in School-Aged Children Study (HBSC) the eating habits and related behaviours of 11-, 13- and 15-year olds were explored in 35 European and North American countries.

The World Health Organization recognises that young people who develop healthy eating habits early in life are more likely to maintain those habits as they mature and to reduce their future risk of chronic diseases such as cardiovascular disease, hypertension, stroke, cancer, non insulin-dependent diabetes and osteoporosis.

Overweight and obesity in young people has been shown to be significantly associated with long-term morbidity and mortality. Strong evidence confirms this link and also suggests that long-term health is compromised by overweight during adolescence, as it is associated with increased mortality especially from coronary heart disease.

Overweight and obesity can be prevented by health eating habits and an adequate level of physical activity.

**Proportion
OVERWEIGHT/OBESE
(15-year olds)**

Percentage ranges:

= 15-27%

= 10-14%

= 4-9%

Source: HBSC research network

Eating habits, body image, weight control and body weight of European young people

There is evidence in the HBSC study to suggest that there is a significant number of young people who do not conform to current nutritional advice. Fruit and vegetable consumption is relatively low and decreases with age. For example the percentage reporting eating fruit on a daily basis ranges from 38% amongst 11-year olds, 33% amongst 13-year olds to 29% amongst 15-year olds. Across age groups girls consistently report eating fruit more than boys.

**Proportion
EATING FRUIT
every day (15-year olds)**

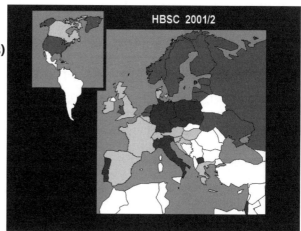

Percentage ranges:

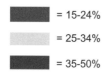

■ = 15-24%

▢ = 25-34%

■ = 35-50%

**Proportion
EATING VEGETABLES
every day) 15-year olds**

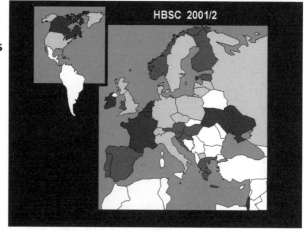

Percentage ranges:

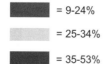

■ = 9-24%

▢ = 25-34%

■ = 35-53%

Source: HBSC research network

A similar pattern exists for the consumption of vegetables. Substantial variation in the consumption of fruit and vegetables exists across countries. The largest differences occur amongst 15-year olds, highlighting a threefold and fivefold gap between the highest and lowest countries reporting daily consumption of fruit and vegetables respectively.

The findings indicate that a high consumption of soft drinks is common among adolescents. About 30% of the students consume soft drinks every day in many countries, more boys than girls of all age groups consume soft drinks on a daily basis.

A significant number of young people skip breakfast. The results for having breakfast every day show great variation between countries, for example ranging from 44% to 89% for 11-year olds. Boys have breakfast more often than girls. The gender difference becomes more pronounced by age.

Body dissatisfaction and dieting are common in both boys and girls, although many more girls report that they think their body is too fat and that they are currently on a diet or believe they need to lose weight. Both behaviours increase steeply with age amongst girls but not with boys. Whilst substantial variation in body dissatisfaction exists between countries, the study shows that at the age of 15, even in the country reporting the lowest prevalence of dieting, well over a third (38%) of girls report that they are on a diet or doing something to lose weight or believe that they need to lose weight.

**Proportion
ON A DIET/TRYING TO
LOSE WEIGHT:
GIRLS (15-year olds)**

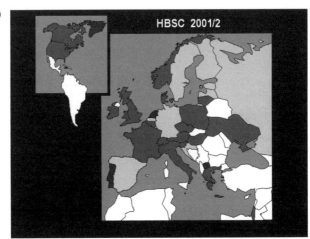

Percentage ranges:

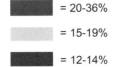

    = 20-36%

    = 15-19%

    = 12-14%

Source: HBSC research network

Self-reported height and weight measurements were used to calculate levels of overweight and obesity among the young people in this study. Whilst caution should be taken in the use of these figures, a number of important observations can be made. Boys are significantly more likely to be overweight than girls in all countries. Overall, about one in six 15-year-old boys are overweight, although this figure rises to over a third of boys in the highest ranking country.

Physical activity and sedentary behaviour

There is a substantial number of young people in all countries who do not meet the current recommended guidelines for physical activity for young people, namely one hour of at least moderate physical activity every day. In almost all countries fewer than half of young people across all age groups report not meeting the guidelines. Activity levels fall steadily with increasing age and the rate of decline is steeper amongst girls. However these figures may mask specific patterns occurring within particular countries. There are wide variations in patterns of physical activity across countries. For example amongst 15-year-olds, the proportion of young people meeting the physical activity guidelines fell from around one in two in the top ranking country to less than one in five the lowest.

Overall, over a quarter of young people were high TV watchers (defined as four or more hours a day), one in seven spent more than three hours a day on the computer and almost one in five spent more than three hours a day during the week doing homework. Patterns of sedentary behaviour also varied considerably across countries. For example amongst 11-year olds there was about a sevenfold difference between the reported levels of high TV watching, a sixfold difference between reported levels of high computer usage and a 17-fold difference in long homework hours during the week. However, all countries demonstrate a consistent gender difference in high PC use and long homework hours. While watching TV and videos is universally popular among both boys and girls, high PC use is more likely among boys and long homework hours are more likely among girls.

Conclusions

From the cross-national data we can conclude that programmes to improve the eating habits and physical activity of young people are strongly needed.

Eating habits and physical activity are influenced by many interacting factors at the individual (e.g. biological, psychological), social (e.g. family and peers), physical environment (e.g. school, sporting facilities) and macro-system or societal level (e.g. mass media, social and cultural norms).

Young people should receive messages from a variety of sources including the school.

Further information

More information on the health behaviour of schoolchildren research can be obtained on the website at www.hbsc.org, or by contacting country co-ordinators. The latest international report was published in February 2004.

Eating at school – A European study

Fannie DE BOER, International Agricultural Centre, Wageningen University, The Netherlands

The following are the extended highlights of a report of the outcomes of a European Survey on issues related to food provision at school, undertaken by the author prior to the forum.

Eating at school – Making healthy choices

Health and good nutritional status are essential for good performance in school and later in life. At the same time an individual's educational level influences health, ability and motivation to maintain a healthy lifestyle. Well-designed and managed nutrition education programmes can, at relatively low costs, alter the nutritional behaviour of schoolchildren. However, very often these programmes do not reflect the provision of food in schools, essential for creating healthy environments in schools. The European Network of Health Promoting Schools (ENHPS) is working towards the integration of health promotion into all aspects of schools.

The present survey was carried out on behalf of the Council of Europe and WHO, Regional Office for Europe as the starting point for this Forum. The survey was held amongst the members of the ENHPS and focuses on exploring the current practices of food provision systems in schools, how this is linked to healthy nutrition within the curriculum and in how far the two are embedded in the whole school approach. The survey is based on an earlier survey in 1997 on 'Healthy Eating for Young People in Europe', published as part of a European Guide by WHO, Regional Office for Europe, 1998. This presentation will highlight the main findings of the new survey.

The objectives for the survey were threefold; firstly, to explore the provision of food in schools across Europe; secondly, to find out how food provision is linked with nutrition education in primary and secondary schools. The third objective dealt with how the provision of food and nutrition education is embedded in the whole school approach.

Topics of the former survey were taken as a basis for the questionnaire. Members of a small task force established for preparation of the Forum were invited to contribute to the selection of the topics. The questionnaire was field tested in Denmark and the Netherlands.

The final questionnaire was sent by the Secretariat of the Council of Europe Ad hoc group to all national co-ordinators of the European Network of Health Promoting Schools, asking them to forward it to experts in the nutrition education field, if necessary. The results I will share with you have to be treated with respect to the limitations of the study. Around half of the countries responded, this is too low a response to generalise results. In certain countries health-promoting activities in schools are decentralised to regional or local level, the questionnaire however asked for data collected at national level. This meant that sometimes reasonable assumptions were made either by the countries or myself, in order to make a comparison between countries possible. Not all data were easily accessible for all respondents so not all questions were answered.

Respondents were: Albania, Belgium, Croatia, Cyprus, Czech Republic, Denmark, France, Finland, Germany, Ireland, Latvia, Lithuania, Luxembourg, Moldavia, the Netherlands, Poland, Portugal, Scotland, Slovakia, Slovenia, Spain, Switzerland, Turkey, Wales and case studies from England. In addition, other countries also returned their questionnaire after the deadline, and unfortunately I could not include their data for this presentation. Their results will be included in my final report.

General results: main nutrition-related health problems

Overweight and its more severe form, obesity, were mentioned in our research by 12 of the 16 countries. The risks related to overweight and the need to design approaches to address this issue was highlighted by Lea Maes in her presentation. Many countries are starting programmes addressing overweight by promoting physical activity and healthy eating. In addition, underweight and its more severe form, malnutrition, was reported by more than half of the countries. The provision of food in schools is of crucial importance for these children. Underweight is not always due to lack of food but can also be caused by severe dieting as is shown in the results of the HBSC study. Malnutrition due to a lack of food was reported more by low-income countries and countries in transition.

Research(1) has shown that children who lack certain nutrients in their diet such as iron and iodine, or who suffer from malnutrition, hunger and parasitic infections, do not have the same potential for learning as do healthy and well-nourished children. Programmes serving a meal during the day or a healthy breakfast could be very beneficial for the cognitive development of these schoolchildren and improve the effectiveness of the educational system. If we want to increase the child's learning at school, more attention should be placed on his/her nutritional well-being.

Policies, rules and regulations

Policies at school level, based on the guidelines for healthy eating are needed to support the provision of food in schools. Policies concerning the hygiene of the food provided are essential to assure safe food.

To the question as to whether there are any nutrition-based regulations for foods served/sold at schools, 17 out of 24 countries responded in the affirmative. In general those regulations were taken from the national healthy eating guidelines.

To the question about regulations concerning hygiene, 20 responded positively, HACCP and Codex Alimentarius were frequently mentioned as examples of these guidelines.

These results indicate that there is more emphasis on food safety in countries than on healthy eating, certainly at the European level. It could also be that regulations on healthy eating are more difficult to develop at the European level or more complex to implement. The question remains of how well these are implemented in schools in the 17 countries that mention national guidelines on healthy eating. Making policies is the first step, but implementing and adhering to them is quite another and some form of inspection/monitoring would seem to be desirable.

In the HBSC survey as well as in this investigation, countries reported a low intake of fruit and vegetables among schoolchildren.

Thirteen countries are now rising to the challenge to improve this and have started special fruit and vegetable programmes for schools, which is an encouraging initiative, especially since this type of initiative was not mentioned in the 1997 survey.[2]

Provision of fruit and vegetables in schools

The majority of these interventions are aimed at primary schools; some of the countries report pilot programmes, offering fruit and vegetables during school breaks as is the case in Belgium, Moldova, the Netherlands, Scotland and Wales. These are often pilot projects for groups of schools in one part of the country, such as in the Netherlands, or already established programmes for all schools like the ones in Scotland and Norway. Some countries serve ample portions of fruit and vegetables as part of the hot meals, as in Lithuania. In the presentation of Norway you will hear more about their intervention concerning implementation of fruit breaks.[4]

Teaching about healthy eating

There is evidence that well-designed and managed nutrition education programmes can, at relatively low cost, alter the nutritional behaviour of schoolchildren.[3] Regarding the question as to whether nutrition was taught in schools,
almost everybody responded positively. However, half said it was not done systematically. Nutrition seems to be taught in many subjects, the most important
ones being science, physical education, health education, and biology. In secondary schools home economics and chemistry are also mentioned.

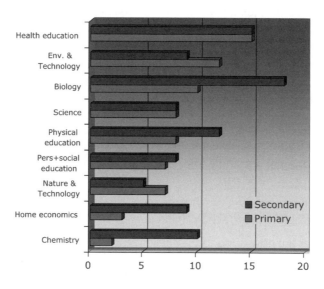

Subjects covering nutrition and food

This outcome is quite similar to the 1997 survey in which subjects such as biology and health education ranked high as a vehicle for nutrition education. How
healthy eating is addressed in these subjects and to what extent other aspects
such as cultural, social, behavioural or lifestyle issues are addressed, we cannot
conclude from the results of this survey. That nutrition education can have an
impact is shown in a poster from Portugal, which reports healthier eating practices among schoolchildren after intensive training.[4]

In primary schools the class teacher is the main source for nutrition education in
schools. For secondary schools the subject teacher is mentioned. But how far are
these teachers trained in nutrition? For primary schools teachers, we see that in

less than half of the countries, teachers are trained in nutrition during their initial training. More countries responded that they had in-service training in nutrition for their teachers.

For secondary schools the response for nutrition during initial teacher training is the same. We might expect that for some subjects like home economics and biology, teachers receive nutrition education as an integrated part of their training. Ideally, there should be more attention for nutrition during initial teacher training courses, especially for primary school teachers. It seems to remain difficult for countries to incorporate this in their teacher training curricula due to time pressures, however it is encouraging that more countries report nutrition to be part of in-service training. A poster from Scotland(4) describes the development of a training manual, which explores the psycho-social issues around healthy eating.

Provision of food in schools

In most countries the provision of food in schools is organised in one way or another although it is not a statutory requirement in all countries. Ways of providing food range from full school meals to providing basic facilities where children can eat their home-brought packed lunch.

For primary schools food is mainly provided in the form of traditional school meal systems or lunchboxes. In addition, special programmes for school milk and fruit and vegetables are common.

In secondary schools there is a wider variety in food provision systems. In addition to the traditional school meals and lunchboxes, students can also get food from cafeterias, vending machines and to a lesser degree from tuck shops.

Special programmes for school milk or fruit and vegetables are not available for these students yet, at least not to any extent. The infrastructure of systems like cafeterias and tuck shops in schools can be used to advantage in introducing programmes selling healthy food such as the fruit tuck shops in Wales. Ines Heindl in her presentation will report on the different food systems which are found in schools in Germany and the guidelines the Germans have developed for these systems.[4]

The existence of vending machines differs considerably between primary and secondary schools. In primary schools, many countries responded that vending machines for soft drinks were not allowed. If they were allowed the majority of these countries responded that they existed only in a small percentage of the schools. For secondary schools we see a much higher presence of soft drinks vending machines. Vending machines for snacks and sweets showed a similar pattern to the one presented for soft drinks.

The introduction of vending machines in schools opens up different issues for debate. Firstly, there is the nutritional point of view. If the vending machine is loaded with high sugar/high fat snacks and sweets and high sugar soft drinks, it will tempt the student in the wrong nutritional direction. In addition, there is the issue of commercial advertisement in schools, an issue over which many nutritionists and health educators express reservations. On the other hand, sales from vending machines may generate additional income for the school. These issues could be turned in a more positive direction. Vending machines as well as cafeterias and tuck shops could also offer more healthy food products, as in the UK for example, where vending machines are stocked with water and other healthy drinks instead of the fizzy ones. In Switzerland they have the Pausen kiosk where students can choose from healthy foods, often organically grown.

With these approaches we might be able to reverse the high intake of simple carbohydrates and offer students the opportunity to select healthier foods during the breaks. Taking into account that 13 of the 19 respondents mentioned high intakes of soft drinks and sugar to be one of the main problems for schoolchildren, this type of programme is definitely needed.

Food planning and food preparation

Student and parent participation in planning meals together with kitchen staff or an external caterer is recommended in a whole school approach, since it creates a wider base for acceptance of the food served or ownership of the choices made. In some countries nutrition action teams or SNAGS (school nutrition action groups) form committed partnerships in schools to facilitate this approach.

Regarding the question as to how meal planning was organised, the majority of countries reported the involvement of either external caterers or school kitchen staff. Five countries mentioned that students had an active part in the preparation of food, namely Denmark, Ireland, the Netherlands, Slovakia and Switzerland. For the Netherlands this is done in special food preparation classes.

A poster from Denmark[4] reports a good example of the involvement of schoolchildren in making choices concerning food, healthy eating and environment.

School food subsidies

Subsidies can be given at national, regional, local or school level. Many countries mentioned that low funding was a major barrier for implementing healthy nutrition in schools. Subsidies for food provision could be an incentive to start such programmes.

In our research 10 countries mentioned that daily meals are subsidised for all children such as in Finland, Spain and Poland. For example in Finland municipalities are responsible for education and receive funds from the national budget to do this. In addition, municipalities collect local taxes, which are used for education, including the provision of meals in schools. Some countries only subsidise meals for socio-economically disadvantaged groups like in Lithuania.

Special programmes such as school milk or fruit and vegetable programmes are subsidised in 12 countries. For example, in the Netherlands the free fruit and vegetable provision for primary schools is subsidised by the European Union, the Ministry of Health and the fruit and vegetables producers. These responses might not reflect hidden subsidies, such as the time and costs of food preparation, kitchen maintenance and other overhead costs, which do not always form a part of the meal costs.

Whole school approach

A health promoting school approach creates a supportive environment for healthier living in which education is linked with healthy eating. This approach is often reflected in a written school health policy.

Sixteen countries mentioned that they have written health policies in primary schools. Of these, 15 mentioned that nutrition is included in the health policy. Eleven countries mentioned that they have these policies in less than 25% of primary schools, for example Ireland, Germany, the Czech Republic, and Belgium, French speaking Community. Five countries are in the 75 - 100% range - Albania, Cyprus, Croatia, Slovakia and Spain.

For secondary schools, 16 countries reported written school health policies, the majority of these fall within the less than 25% of schools category, some in the 75-100% category. Of these, 15 countries reported that nutrition is part of written policies. The question remains, however, how well are these policies implemented?

Gillian Kynoch will report on a new initiative in Scotland where a school meal approach is integrated into a health promoting school approach.

Public/private partnerships

A contract between commercial or private food providers and public schools may have been viewed in the past as a kind of partnership or more as a commissioner/supplier relationship. Nowadays, a partnership implies more: different stakeholders are working together to provide healthy food in school, also at the level of regional or local authority. Compared with the 1997 survey, partnerships have been developing into a more continuing relationship. In 1997 only one-way activities such as supplying educational materials or occasionally supporting special events were described. In our survey, 10 countries reported that there were public/private partnerships in schools, for example Belgium, Denmark, Germany, Switzerland, and Portugal. Examples of these forms of co-operation are: external caterers in Denmark; farmers' wives selling sandwiches, fruit and vegetables in schools in Switzerland; local producers supplying fruit in schools in Belgium and Scotland; national fruit and vegetable producers supplying primary schools in the Netherlands, and milk drinks provided by companies in Slovakia. These partnerships can even extend to schools being built with private funding according to the specifications of the local council, as was reported by Scotland.

Evaluation

Monitoring and evaluation are important tools to show what is successful and what not in healthy nutrition in schools. In the survey we asked what type of evaluations are undertaken in the different countries concerning eating at school and at which level.

Most countries report interventions to be evaluated at national or at school level, less so at regional or local level. Only one country, Luxembourg, reported that they use baseline, process, outcome, impact evaluation and monitoring at the national level. Five countries report baseline studies at national level, and three at regional level (Denmark, Portugal, and Belgium, French speaking Community), one at both, three at local level. Six countries report that they have baseline evaluation in school interventions. Nine countries do not report having any structurally evaluated interventions. It will be important for us to reflect on the barriers for evaluation and monitoring of healthy food provision and to share good practice between countries at this event.

Barriers

Only three countries stated that they did not have any barriers for the implementation of food provision programmes, including monitoring and evaluation. Other countries mentioned the following as the main barriers.

At the individual/school level, countries stated that the following were barriers:

- low priority for healthy nutrition;
- unsupportive school environments towards healthy nutrition;
- school staff who were unmotivated or too overburdened to give attention to healthy nutrition;
- inadequate monitoring and evaluation, partly due to low priority, partly to lack of knowledge on how to set up efficient monitoring and evaluation systems.

At community/national level, countries stated that the following were barriers:

- lack of political will, and the need to convince politicians and other leaders to facilitate healthy nutrition in schools;
- poverty was mentioned quite frequently - families with low financial resources cannot afford to pay for food provided in the schools;
- lack of funding for the schools themselves to implement programmes promoting healthy choices of food in schools;
- monitoring and evaluation are not seen as essential.

Challenges

- to motivate schoolchildren, parents, teachers and other school staff, community members and politicians to focus on healthy eating in schools;
- to address overweight and obesity issues in schoolchildren by designing interventions on the provision of a healthy school environment and good nutrition education that promotes healthy food choices and physical activity;
- to match the taught curriculum on healthy nutrition with the whole school approach. This is what we might previously have called the hidden curriculum, but it is perhaps now time to expose or reveal the hidden curriculum and to demonstrate its importance;
- to establish partnerships to promote healthy food choices in schools;
- to design simple, practical and participatory monitoring and evaluation systems for food provision in schools.

References

1. World Bank – www.wbln0018.worldbank.org

2. Healthy Eating for Young People in Europe; WHO 1998

3. WHO. WHO Information Series on School Health; Healthy Nutrition WHO/SCHOOL/98.4 Geneva. 1998

4. European Forum on Eating at School – Making Healthy Choices Poster Abstracts and Presentations

Participants' interviews

The rapporteur, Ian Young, interviewed a small number of delegates at the event. Here are extracts from some of the personal views expressed

Aileen Robertson, WHO, specialist on nutrition. – The policy context

Rapporteur: How do you see the wider nutrition policy context from WHO perspective – how might that impact on the work we're doing on health promoting schools in Europe?

Aileen: First of all if we start with WHO Headquarters in Geneva, there are several things happening that help to push nutrition much higher up the political agenda.

EUROPE

Deaths in 2000 attributable to selected learning risk factors

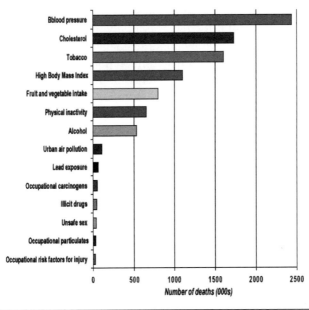

Source: WHR 2002

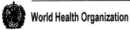
World Health Organization

One thing is the World Health Report 2002, which included the summary of the second analysis of the burden of the global disease. The first global report came out in 1996 and it showed that tobacco and alcohol were major risk factors but nutrition was not mentioned. I believe that now the World Health Report 2002 will do the same thing for nutrition as it did for tobacco in the 1990s, that is, push the issue to the top of the agenda. As a follow-on to that, there is a technical series report (TSR 916) that is being produced jointly by WHO and FAO on the prevention of chronic diseases. It's not necessarily saying anything new, just reinforcing the message of reducing fat, salt, sugar and increasing fruit and vegetables. But what it does is present a comprehensive scientific basis for dietary guidelines with a rubber stamp from scientific experts. A new document 'Global Strategy on Diet, Physical Activity and Health' is being rolled out by WHO Headquarters and it will now be coming to the World Health Assembly of WHO in May 2004. (See appendix 3.)

As part of the global strategy there is now a new initiative on promoting fruit and vegetable consumption in conjunction with FAO.

At a European regional level the regional committee of Euro in 2000 endorsed a resolution on the impact of nutrition on public health and an action plan for the region. This is the first time that nutrition has been on the political agenda in Europe – the work to get it there was not easy. This Action Plan is based on three pillars – nutrition, food safety and a sustainable food supply. This means that countries have to develop national nutrition policies based on this concept. In 2006 there will be a ministerial conference on nutrition policy and this will have two basic aims. One is to assess what impact the European Action Plan endorsed in 2000 has had and how far countries have gone with implementation, and the second thing is that we will develop a strategy policy document for 2006 to 2010.

Rapporteur: That is really helpful to get the policy context from your perspective at WHO, Aileen. Do you have any personal reflections on what schools can contribute to the promotion of healthy eating? We have lots of research on young people's knowledge suggesting that in western European countries, it is relatively good. For example, if you ask 12-year-old students in Scotland what constitutes a healthy diet they can tell you about low sugar, low fat, low salt, higher dietary fibre (90% understand that). Like other countries we have good knowledge levels but in Scotland we have some of the highest sugar consumption in Europe in sweets etc. How do we bridge that gap between knowledge and behaviour in schools and in other settings?

Aileen: It is clearly complex and there are many different factors. There's no doubt that education in nutrition is not going to be successful on its own so there has to be some involvement by the children as a learning experience in terms of food. In a way food doesn't have a value in Europe any more, it's not really valued in the sense it was 50 years ago. So the idea that we should have clean water and fresh air is valued but the fact that we should have good value quality food is not valued in the same way. We have this idea that we want cheaper and cheaper food – but good food costs and we need to learn this. We are now spending only around 10% of our income on food, which is ridiculous – it can't be any less than that otherwise we're only buying food that's mass produced and often high in fat, sugar and salt. The whole value system around food has to be re-thought. It is a society's problem – one of the areas I am interested in is to link the whole idea of the food chain and food production and one aspect is how children can learn where food comes from and how food is planted and grown. I'm not suggesting everyone becomes self-sufficient in producing food but there has to be a better understanding of the importance of food in our society, whether it is local, regional, national or international.

Rapporteur: Another delegate said they should also know how processed food is produced.

Aileen: That whole concept about where food comes from and how it gets there is also to do with consumerism, ethics, fair trade, environmental pollution, pesticides, nitrates – consumer issues about GM foods, and organic foods.

Rapporteur: Do you see popular issues such as organic foods and genetically modified foods which get a lot of publicity in some countries as a side issue to the main thrust of what we're trying to do?

Aileen: Yes it's often the side issues which appear in the media but if we look at the fundamental issues about food I would like to see children have access from a very young age to school gardens or school orchards or some sort of community-related activity like that; they could also visit farms. As a second issue we should try, like the Slovenians, to encourage food to be bought from the local producers. Local authorities could try to have a contract with local producers especially for meat with less fat, milk with less fat, more fruit and vegetables. Local producers would get the business, thus supporting local communities, providing local jobs and also trying to up the brakes on cheap imported food that is high in fat, sugar and salt. My feeling is that there is an awareness that we have to change, especially with regard to the obesity epidemic. People are asking why is this happening. So it's about looking at our value system and asking where does food fit in with this value system and how can we address the future.

Sara Hunter, aged 15, from Plockton High School, Scotland – Young Minds

Rapporteur: Has the Young Minds project made an impact on your school?

Sara: I can honestly say the biggest change in the school, and carried on outside school, is drinking water – no one appears to drink fizzy drinks anymore. Most people enjoy the new healthy options, which have been included in the menu, and everyone buys the cereal bars and goes to the breakfast club. Whether they do it outside I'm not sure but definitely in the school.

Rapporteur: In terms of the international dimension, what are the benefits?

Sara: You see different cultures e.g. we're not allowed to eat in our classrooms but the Danish people are, they also call their teacher by their first name and don't wear uniforms!

Maria Haukrogh, Danish Food Administration. – Involving Consumers

Rapporteur: Maria can you tell me about changes happening in Denmark in food provision in schools?

Maria: One thing I would like to highlight and that is the way the Danish Government has chosen to establish a scheme where it is the intention that the initiative comes from the consumers. The schools and institutions are encouraged to contact us if they want any help.

The main goal in this project is to encourage schools to create or to establish meals in schools at different levels. For example, small tuck shop or canteen with meal. The success of this depends on the use of the school, the parents and the board. The second thing is that we have tried a regional approach where we have 11 districts in Denmark where one person working on this has a close relationship with the schools in the different counties or districts where they work part-time. They have contact with the schools where they go out and make contact when they've had a call on the hot line. They set up a meeting with the board and we follow it up. It's better to do this on a regional level rather than a national level. We have an educational scheme where we have 11 working days where people have been trained to use this consultancy approach and where we try to find out what's important for the people concerned.

Rapporteur: Explain the consultancy role as opposed to the nutritional role. Do they have any formal qualifications or are they working on a practical level?

Maria: It could be the home economics teacher or a parent or whoever thinks this is important and they want to make a difference. It's not people who are nutritionists.

Rapporteur: There is no tradition in Denmark of providing schools meals – one survey suggested that 25% of young people in Copenhagen were coming to school without any food. Is that fairly typical or is it higher in a big city?

Maria: Of course Copenhagen has a higher level but it is an issue that young people don't eat breakfast and then they don't take lunch maybe twice a week. That means it is a big issue in Denmark that kids don't get fed in schools.

Rapporteur: Is this an issue in modern life with family life not always conforming to traditional norms?

Maria: It's also that kids are spending maybe 70% of their time outside the home so they go away at 7.30 in the morning and come home at five in the evening. It is important that we create environments in schools and elsewhere to help young people get accessibility to good food or what we think is reasonable to eat.

Jenny Woolfe, Food Standards Agency, United Kingdom – Developing Skills

Rapporteur: Jenny, you mentioned the development of skills that young people could use as a part of living independently?

Jenny: Yes, I spoke about this in one of the discussion sessions. I believe that if young people are to eat more healthily they need to understand what constitutes a healthy diet and have the practical skills to put this knowledge into practice. The Food Standards Agency UK (FSA) has convened a cross-Government group, which includes Department for Education and Skills (DfES), Department of Health, Health Development Agency, Qualifications and Curriculum Authority, Design and Technology Association (DATA), and Children & Young People's Unit to collaborate on this initiative. The aim is to compare the skills and abilities of 14 to 16-year-olds against a range of core competencies, which have been identified under the main themes of diet and health, consumer awareness, food preparation and handling skills and food hygiene and safety.

Qualitative fieldwork with focus groups and friendship pairs of young people from the target age group was commissioned to investigate what young people already know and can do and where the gaps are that need to be addressed. The report of this work is available on the Agency website at www.food.gov.uk/multimedia/pdfs/competencyevaluation.pdf

A joint FSA/DfES public consultation 'Getting to Grips with Grub' sought views on the nature of the competencies identified by the steering group and means of delivering them locally in a sustainable way. The Agency has also sought the views of young people through the National Children's Bureau. The results will be collated, summarised and published on the Agency's website.

Introduction

The Young Minds approach is based on a view that young people can develop shared visions and actions which transcend national boundaries and it utilises information and communications technology (ICT) to facilitate this process. The approach was first developed at the 8th meeting of national co-ordinators for The European Network of Health Promoting Schools (ENHPS) in 2000 and it was extended at the conference Education and Health in Partnership, in Egmond, the Netherlands in 2002. The approach is based on the view that students' action competence, or the ability to take reflective action and bring about positive change with reference to health, is central to the learning process. In addition to the presentations in the lecture hall, the Young Minds project provided an inter-active dimension to the forum both for participants who were physically at the event and for others who had an electronic presence through email.

Young Minds at the forum

The Young Minds project worked on specific issues on healthy eating in schools at the forum. In addition to the pupils and teachers present from Denmark, Scot-land and the Netherlands, there was considerable electronic dialogue with school pupils in Spain.

Various IT dialogues took place at the event and these are listed below:

1. dialogue between external teachers and the chairman of the conference
2. dialogue between external teachers and keynote speaker at the conference
3. dialogue between external teachers and teachers at the conference
4. dialogue between external students and students internal to the conference
5. a triangular dialogue: two external (1 student, 1 adult) and one internal student.

An example of each category is given below.

1. Dialogue between Spanish teachers and Bent Mikkelsen

Author: Chary and Espe, teachers, Spain

Date: 11/20/2003 2:11:38 PM

Subject: a suggestion for joint action

Message: Hi everybody,
We are two teachers from Spain and we think that there should be a nutritional committee to design a common document that all European countries would be able to use together. Of course this document should be adapted to each partic-ular country and also families should be taken into account.

* * * * * * * * * * * * * * *

Author: Bent Egberg Mikkelsen

Date: 11/20/2003 3:50:01 PM

Subject: RE: a suggestion for joint action

Message: Hello teachers,
A European document is actually what is in on our minds. And you are right it should be adapted nationally. We will probably end up with recommendations and practical guidelines in the near future.

Bent Egberg Mikkelsen
Chairman of the forum

2. Dialogue between Spanish teachers and speaker, F. De Boer

Author: Rachel, teacher, Spain

Date: 11/20/2003 4:06:39 PM

Subject: to Mrs Fannie De Boer on Eating at School

Message: As teachers we have seen how, in the last two decades, almost 100% of the food facilities in Spanish schools changed from being run by the same schools to industrial and private enterprises.
We wonder about the consequences of this shift.
Should this activity be ruled under other aims than profit?
We are waiting for your opinion. Thank you. Best wishes from Alcalá

* * * * * * * * * * * * * * *

Author: Fannie de Boer

Date: 11/20/2003 5:53:03 PM

Subject: RE: to Mrs Fannie de Boer on Eating at School

Message: Dear Rachel
Many thanks for your question.
I do not think it is bad in principle if you change from school paid caterers to private enterprise. In general you can control them better. However, it all depends on what they serve, what kind of policies you do to ensure healthy food.
Your last question is quite interesting. I agree with you it should not be only profit aimed. I think it is quite important to have also other types of considerations

involved with the provision of food, it should be safe, healthy but also affordable for all the people who like to use it. If it only will be on maximising the profits, it will fall short on all what we are talking about here.

Take care and saludos de Strasbourg. Fannie

3. Dialogue between Spanish teachers and Young Mind teachers at the conference

Author: Maria José, teacher, Spain

Date: 11/20/2003 4:34:58 PM

Subject: We have to leave the forum for today

Message: Hi!
We have to leave you for today, but we'll keep in touch and follow up tomorrow what you have done today.
As you have seen, two more colleagues have participated and also some students of other grades who were familiar with YM.
We have had great fun and that is also very important for our health, isn't it?

Have a good evening and keep us in mind!

* * * * * * * * * * * * * * *

Author: Donald Ferguson, Young Minds Teacher, Scotland

Date: 11/20/2003 6:07:39 PM

Subject: RE: We have to leave the forum for today

Message: Hola Maria,
Donald here.
I am in Strasbourg with a colleague from home economics, Catriona, and also two pupils, Sara, whom you met last year, and a new girl, Tara.
We have been looking in a workshop at ways of involving parents, politicians, and local authorities in the issue of healthy eating and getting them to take it seriously. We have come up with the following ideas:

1. sending letters to politicians detailing the damage to health caused by unwholesome food, and an outline of statistics of other countries and the consequences drawn from them by these countries;

2. inviting local newspapers to interview pupils about eating habits, and high-lighting concerns – also inviting these newspapers to feature successful school ventures into wholesome eating;

3. inviting school boards to discuss issues of nutrition so that there is parental involvement;

4. using school-based projects to bring parents in or otherwise influence them in the direction of healthy eating;

5. getting the government to target parents about the dangers of unwholesome food and to provide information on how to quickly prepare healthy meals for children;

6. ensuring that there are democratic forums in schools – Youth Board etc. – so that pupils can target parents, local authorities, and politicians with letters, recommendations, and suggestions for action.

Let us know what you think. Muchas gracias,

Cheerio,
Donald

4. Dialogue between students internal and external to the conference

Author: Kaija, Denmark

Date: 11/18/2003 11:18:53 AM

Subject: Food at your school

Message: Dear Spain.
We would like to know, what you think about the food at your school.
And how you like it to be. So can we tell about it too.

Thank you.
From Kasper, Käthe, and Kaija

* * * * * * * * * * * * * * *

Author: Rakel, 2°A, Spain

Date: 11/20/2003 3:13:53 PM

Subject: RE: Food at your school

Message: I guess we do not have bad food, but it is not good enough! we have every kind of sandwiches but there are no fruit, juices (just sodas) or salads. I would like to have more choices, and also to create a really healthy environment,

because it is not banned to smoke at our cafeteria, and that makes me sick! The most days I have to go downtown and miss my whole break time.
Does it help you? I hope so,

Rakel.

* * * * * * * * * * * * * * *

Author: Pilar, Spain

Date: 11/20/2003 12:32:22 PM

Subject: RE: Food at your school

Message: Dear Kaija, Kasper and Kathe,
I'm Pilar, one of the participants in the YM project on Alcohol, Youth and Culture. I am writing with my class mate Carlos (1a bachillerato G).
We do not have a proper canteen at our school, only a cafeteria where we can buy food which is not too healthy (buns, pastries, sandwiches, industrial snacks, soft drinks, coffee, etc.). It is very expensive and some people go out and buy their mid-morning snack in the shops around school; other people bring their food from home.
We think that should change because it is very important that we can find healthy and cheap food easily in our school.
Would you mind to send us some ideas about to approach this problem?

* * * * * * * * * * * * * * *

Author: Kaija, Denmark

Date: 11/20/2003 1:06:58 PM

Subject: RE: RE: Food at your school

Message: Dear Pilar,
Thanks for your answer.
Spain is represented at this conference, and if any decisions are taken, it will probably also be better in Spain.
Or else you can try to talk with your municipality about food at schools, and other places. Like in Ballerup municipality in Denmark, where a student from Maalov school told them that the food was very bad at the school. So they decided that it should be better. You can try to go in at the Danish page, under interview, there you can read something about it.

From Kaija

5. A triangular dialogue

Author: Pilar, Spain

Date: 11/20/2003 3:03:49 PM

Subject: Hi people!!
Message: I'm Pilar, from Spain, I was a student of 1° Bachillerato. I was a participant in the last YM project. It was fantastic because we worked very hard and we
got good results and I think that our lives have changed.
I'm also interested in this new project, and I think that the school's food wasn't
healthy and I would like to work with you in order to have information of the different schools' food and to know how to get good results in this work.
Best wishes.

Pilar

* * * * * * * * * * * * * * *

Author: taz

Date: 11/21/2003 9:04:37 AM

Subject: RE: Hi people!!
Message: Hi Pilar its Sara and Tara from Scotland! Sara was at the conference last
year and I was part of the home team. We also think that our lives have been
altered by the conference.

* * * * * * * * * * * * * * *

Author: Venka (Young Minds facilitator)

Date: 11/21/2003 9:20:17 AM

Subject: RE: RE: Hi people!!
Message: Hi there,
Can you explain a bit more, how the conference and the project altered your
lives? I would really be happy to hear more about that, as I was involved in last
year's Young Minds…

* * * * * * * * * * * * * * *

Author: taz

Date: 11/21/2003 9:44:28 AM

Subject: RE: RE: RE: Hi people!!

Message: Well after the conference we decided to institute more healthy options in our school. We got rid of all the fizzy drinks and replaced them with water and fruit juices. We replaced the sweets with healthy fruit bars and fresh fruit salads. This has made our lives healthier and makes us feel and look better.

The teachers' voices in the Young Minds project

1. Teachers share their visions on healthy eating with pupils.

2. Pupils make their own suggestions and are allowed to action them.

3. Teachers empower pupils immediately (the pupils' future is now) if pupils wish to initiate a food change. Even if it means spending money.

4. Pupils must be allowed to explore 'cool' options to make healthy eating credible to their peers.

5. Teachers support pupils through the learning experience – through all classroom subjects – pupils should have democratic opportunities through their committees, and also in impromptu classroom discussions.

6. Initiatives can be political (Scotland) or communal (community and students) (Denmark)

7. The dynamics of education – empower children democratically early (in primary school) to make healthy eating changes in the school.

8. Television and commercial companies present a hurdle because they promote what makes money for them. Organic and local food suppliers can be contacted to supply school canteens.

9. If children get a chance to develop their ideas internationally as in 'Young Minds' then they can influence the future in favour of healthy eating.

Catriona Ferguson, Donald Ferguson, Käthe Bruun Jensen, Pyt Jon Sikkema.

The students' common vision

Young Minds reported back on their work during the forum, and described their poster exhibition and pyramid, showing visions of 'food at school'. In the period prior to the conference, the students from Denmark, the Netherlands and Scotland collaborated, using the Internet, on developing their shared vision on the topic 'food at school.'

The following is a quotation of the vision espoused by Young Minds students as a result of their forum discussions.

"This is the common vision that we have come up with.

We think that lunch at school should be served in one big dining room with music played. You should be able to sit there the entire lunch time if you wish, allowing you to enjoy your food and take your time over it!! The food should be set out in the form of a buffet (you know, like in hotels) thus covering a wide range of food that doesn't necessarily have to be all healthy. Some could be stodgy so pupils learn to make the right decisions themselves!! There should also be a new foreign food everyday so food is varied and more exciting!! Pupils should also be allowed to request favourite meals, so that they are participating in the decisions!

We also think that fruit and water should be given out free in each class and be allowed to be consumed during the lessons. It should also be made compulsory that healthy eating lessons are given to all students, the way in Scotland physical education is compulsory. This means pupils are learning about the importance of food choice as well as putting the methods into practice, hopefully encouraging pupils to take healthy eating beyond the school walls and into the world, teaching others, and most importantly bringing up their children to do the same.

We think that students should 'work' as canteen helpers, and they should be educated in healthiness."

Is there a healthy school meal?

Ines HEINDL, Universität Flensburg, Germany

These are the highlights of a presentation, in which Ines Heindl explores the breadth of aesthetic, psychological, social and cultural issues, as well as the role of education and the whole school, in promoting healthy eating.

Nutrition education and its importance

Nutrition – what people eat – is known to be one of the key factors influencing health. If people eat healthily, they can avoid many preventable diseases and can live longer lives with fewer illnesses. Many European countries have attempted to introduce campaigns for healthier eating, and there is widespread concern about the trend towards a fast-food culture in which traditional styles of eating and cooking are declining (Dixey et al. 1999).

Whereas health professionals can clearly see the relationship between diet and health, most people's diet and food preferences are determined more by social, economic, climatic and geographical factors and by religion and customs than by concern for health. In Europe's rich cultural diversity food and eating are powerful expressions of cultural and social identity, and this is a factor that must be taken into account in any attempt to encourage people to eat healthily. Even in Europe many people do not have enough money to provide themselves and their families with a healthy diet. Nutrition education, therefore, needs to consider all these issues, including the cultural and financial ones (Dixey et al. 1999).

In order to be effective, nutrition education must:

- be personally relevant;
- be clearly understandable;
- use food and meals rather than nutrients as a conceptual basis;
- be consistent in dietary messages;
- take into account people's perception of relative risks;
- emphasise the benefits of change;
- address the barriers of making dietary changes.

Nutrition and health for young people

Main health problems for adults in the European Union are obesity, cardiovascular diseases and cancer. The Kiel Obesity Prevention Study (KOPS), one of the most important research projects in Germany, which started in 1996 and will end 2009, is looking at obesity in childhood. First results clearly reveal the following facts (Müller et al. 2001; Müller 2002; Danielzik 2003):

- compared to results of 1978, 23% of the five to seven-year-old children and 40% of the nine to 11-year-old children are overweight;

- those children are more often found in families with obese parents, low income and a low social status (school-leaving certificates of their parents). Obese children try to avoid physical activities more often than other children;

- children with low interest in physical activities from families with a low social status spend more time in front of television, videos, computers and tend to prefer fast food, snacks, chips, fat sausages, sweets, fizzy drinks, etc. Beyond this, there is no general connection between the quality of nutrition and obesity.

The organisers of the Kiel Prevention Study are not satisfied with simply presenting these new research data. Professor Müller and his team also offer support programmes to schools and families and evaluate acceptance and efficacy. After five years of intervention there are obvious signs of success in the schools concerned, but families with obese children seem to take only marginal interest in this project. Only 20% of all the parents the Kiel project tried to get involved are participating and willing to co-operate.

According to Professor Müller and the WHO, obesity starting in childhood is at present the most urgent health problem ('obesity epidemic'). Prevention programmes seem to highlight the fact that interventions may have an influence on the incidence of obesity, but not on its persistence. It has, moreover, become evident that the crisis of our health system is an unrecognised crisis of our education system.

Germany after the Programme for International Student Assessment (PISA)

The health and nutrition problems in Germany can be connected to the changing situation in schools after PISA. The Germans fairly quickly responded to the bad results compared to other European countries as part of the PISA study. Not only schools but also parents were made responsible for the lack of education, missing support of children to develop strategies for life-long learning. The

German school system is, by and large, one of half-time schools, which is now supposed to be turned into one of all-day schools. The German federal government offers an investment programme with a target of 10,000 all-day schools. At first glance the new concepts seem to be considering everything for better learning conditions. The facilities for healthy meals in all-day schools, however, are often considered to be purely organisational problems, a view taken by school authorities and sometimes by heads too. Financial considerations are prevalent, and it is often the cheapest offers from caterers that are accepted.

Even at the time of the predominantly half-day school system in Germany it did not seem legitimate to adopt the view that the school was responsible only for feeding children's minds, or put differently: German schools only provided food for thought. Young people and teachers who stay and work at school all day long can expect ideas and concepts that include both mind and body as well as social and cultural issues. School-related projects on Health Promotion (European Network of Health Promoting Schools) all around Europe are already in existence: so nobody has to start from scratch.

The school-based nutrition education guide 'Healthy eating for young people in Europe' (Dixey et al. 1999) consists of a planned and sequential core curriculum. What is offered to children, either within the classroom or as part of the whole school experience, needs to be planned and co-ordinated appropriate to their developmental stages. This is a sound educational principle, but health education and nutrition education are often not co-ordinated across school. The idea of a spiral curriculum, as part of the guide, involves repeating and extending the work on a topic in a dialectical fashion as children develop.

A health-promoting school concerned with nutrition education would be expected to :

- have nutrition teaching that is provided by adequate resources;
- develop a statement of policy about nutrition education;
- focus on enjoyment of food;
- promote training for staff, teachers, caterers and cleaners, in healthy eating;
- provide comfortable surroundings in which children and staff can enjoy eating;
- enable healthy choices if food is provided at the school;
- involve parents and the wider community;
- be explicitly concerned that no child is hungry while at school and that poor nutrition does not affect learning;

- co-ordinate all aspects of nutrition education to ensure efficient use of resources and to minimise contradictory messages;
- ensure that all staff are committed to the goals of the health-promoting school and be explicitly concerned about the health and well-being of both pupils and staff. *(Stockley 1993)*.

The Netherlands, Portugal and Spain have implemented this guide through materials and policies. Since legislation and administration in the field of education predominantly fall within the scope of the individual German states, the process of implementation takes longer, but a promising start has been made (Heindl 2003).

Meals at school should be balanced in nutrients

Demands for wholesome meals at school led to recommendations for rules and regulations in Germany, but not every local government has transformed them yet into policies. Lower Saxony and Saxony-Anhalt have implemented specific regulations, and North Rhine-Westphalia formulated recommendations on breaks and meals at schools, as a right for pupils and staff.

The German Society of Nutrition (DGE) set up a working group of experts on nutrition in schools, with specific instructions to focus on eating times and food and nutrition quality at school. Two recent publications on nutrition in all-day schools demonstrate the urgency (Heseker et al. 2003a,b) of supporting recommendations.

The expert group distinguishes between different catering systems, as there are:
- freshly prepared meals by a kitchen staff at school, responsibility of different authorities (also parent organisations);
- distribution system (preparation of meals in an external kitchen);
- processing or regeneration system (i.e. cook and chill-food);
- a mixture of different systems (i.e. externally pre-prepared main courses completed by salads and deserts at school);
- extended food choices at kiosks;
- fast food systems (i.e. fast food restaurants supply meals);
- cold meals systems.

Furthermore the expert group comments on these different systems to enable schools to make informed decisions. As might have been expected, freshly prepared food at school has all the advantages of a wholesome meal, because of its sensual, nutritional and social values: attractive meals within attractive surroundings, flexible response to the wishes of the customers, no restriction on the choice of food for those who prepare the meals, daily communication between kitchen staff, teachers and pupils. But it is also known that quality is not the only factor one has to take into account, and often there seem to be economic reasons against freshly prepared food in schools. Carefully prepared fresh food also needs qualified kitchen staff. When comparing the different possible catering systems, acceptable compromises between hot and cold meals should be made on the basis of demands for the physical, mental, intellectual and social efficiency of pupils, teachers and other members of staff.

The criteria for these demands are:

- sensual quality: smell, taste, consistency, colour etc. of meals;
- nutritional quality: ratio of nutrients for a wholesome and healthy nutrition;
- learning processes: positively affected by wholesome food;
- messages: compatibility with both classroom and general school issues;
- decision-making: promoting healthy choices when considering different offers;
- eating atmosphere: enjoyable meals, pleasant eating places;
- participation: influence on the catering system by the customers.

Aesthetic and cultural issues of a healthy school meal

Young children can learn to enjoy almost every food, hot and spicy food, bland healthy food, fast food, depending on what people around them eat (Schlosser 2002). The different cultures of the world support the view that meals that are supposed to set the standards have to be sensually attractive to children and should be enjoyed in a positive atmosphere. The human sense of smell is still not fully understood and can greatly be affected by psychological factors and expectations. The colour of food can determine the perception of its taste. The mind filters out the overwhelming majority of aromas that surround us, focusing intently on some, ignoring others. People can get accustomed to bad smells or good smells. A smell can suddenly evoke a long forgotten moment. The flavours of childhood food seem to leave an indelible mark, and adults often return to them, sometimes without knowing why. These 'comfort foods' become a source of pleasure and reassurance (Hirschfelder 2001), a fact fast food chains work hard to promote.

Childhood memories of 'Happy Meals' can translate into a chance for parents and school catering. Why not try to learn from fast food restaurants? Their success is mainly built on product binding through flavour, typical combination of foods in an unconventional atmosphere and added values (toys, games etc.). Kindergarten children and primary schoolchildren in particular want to know what their meals consist of, and they take a keen interest in foods, smells, tastes and consistencies. Sensual education through food and meals at school would create those happy memories in a socially positive atmosphere.

Bibliography and further reading

Danielzik, S. (2003). *Epidemiologie von Übergewicht und Adipositas bei Kindern in Kiel: Daten der ersten Querschnittuntersuchung der Kieler Adipositas-Präventionsstudie* (Kiel Obesity Prevention Study). Universität Kiel: Dissertation.

Dixey, R., Heindl, I., Loureiro I., Pérez-Rodrigo, C., Snel, J., und Warnking, P. (1999). *Healthy eating for young people in Europe – a school-based nutrition education guide.* WHO.

Heindl, Ines (2003). *Studienbuch Ernährungsbildung – Ein europäisches Konzept zur schulischen Gesundheitsförderung (Study book Nutrition Education – a European concept of Health Promotion at school).* Bad Heilbrunn: Klinkhardt Verlag.

Heseker, H., Beer, S., Schlegel-Matthies, K., Heindl, I., und Methfessel, B. (2003a). *Ernährung in der Ganztagsschule. Teil 1: Notwendigkeit und Problematik von Schulverpflegung.* In: Ernährungsumschau 50 (3), pp B9-12.

Heseker, H., Beer, S., Schlegel-Matthies, K., Heindl, I., und Methfessel, B. (2003b). *Ernährung in der Ganztagsschule. Teil 2: Institutionalisierung und Möglichkeiten von Schulverpflegung.* In: Ernährungsumschau 50 (4), pp B13-16.

Hirschfelder, G. (2001). *Europäische Esskultur – Geschichte der Ernährung von der Steinzeit bis heute.* Frankfurt: Campus Verlag.

Müller, M.J., Mast, M., und Langnäse, K. (2001). *Werden wir eine Gesellschaft der Dicken?* Münchner Medizinische Wochenschrift 28, pp 863-867.

Müller, J. (2002). *Wie erfolgreich ist Ernährungserziehung im Vor- und Grundschulalter?* Tagungsband zum 5. aid-Forum. aid Special, pp 27-28.

Murcott, A. (2003). *Food and Culture.* In: P.S. Belton and T. Belton (Eds.) (2003). *Food, Science and Society – Exploring the gap between expert advice and individual behaviour.* Berlin: Springer Verlag, pp 21-53.

Schlosser, E. (2002). *Fast Food Nation – the dark side of the all-american meal.* New York: Perennial edition.

Stockley, L. (1993). *The promotion of healthier eating: a basis for action.* London: Health Education Authority.

Hungry for success:
A whole approach to school meals in scotland

Gillian Kynoch, Scottish Food and Health Co-ordinator, Scottish Executive Health Department

These are the extended highlights of Gillian Kynoch's presentation describing how The Scottish Executive has invested in a revitalised school meals service in Scotland with nutritional standards being developed for school meals.

Introduction

In January 2002, Scottish Ministers established an Expert Panel on School Meals to make recommendations that would form the framework of a national strategy for school meals. The Panel's remit was to provide cost recommendations and a fully developed implementation strategy to:

• establish standards for school meals;

• improve the presentation of school meals to improve general take-up;

• eliminate any stigma attached to taking free school meals.

In February 2003, Hungry for Success, the report of the Expert Panel on School Meals, was published. This report sets out the Panel's vision for a revitalised school meals service in Scotland and presents a number of far-reaching recommendations. Ministers have accepted all the Panel's recommendations including the national nutrient-based standards for school lunches and they are also seen in the context of health promoting schools in Scotland.

These standards are the first of their kind in the UK. They form a key part of the Scottish Executive's major drive to improve Scotland's health record by improving the nation's diet.

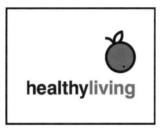

healthyliving

The Scottish Executive's Healthy Living Campaign, shown in the logo above, and the Scottish Diet Action Plan seek to increase the amount of fresh fruit and vegetables in our diet and reduce the high consumption of fat, sugar and salt. These new standards offer the opportunity of achieving major and lasting improvements to the health of Scotland's children by ensuring that our children have access to high-quality school meals.

Local authorities, schools and caterers are being asked to work in partnership with parents and pupils to implement the standards in all primary and special schools by December 2004 and in all secondary schools by December 2006. Later this year the standards will be supplemented by product specifications and nutritional analysis software to aid implementation and monitoring of the standards.

Nutrient-based standards for school meals

Diet in childhood plays an essential role in growth and development, current well-being, educational performance and avoidance of chronic disease throughout life. Current knowledge on optimal diet for children is set out in the 'Dietary Reference Values Report' (1991) for the UK and it is this report that forms the scientific basis for the design of the Scottish Nutrient Standards.

The proportion of the daily nutrient provision that should be achieved from a single daily lunch has been extensively reviewed by the Caroline Walker Trust Expert Working Group on School Meals (1992), the outcome of which were the 'Nutritional Guidelines for School Meals'. These Guidelines cover the nutrients and micronutrients (vitamins and minerals) currently of most concern in schoolchildren's diets and remain largely appropriate for calculating the nutrient standards for Scottish schoolchildren. They were therefore adopted as the basis of the recommended nutrient standards. In addition,

- fruit and vegetables are considered as part of the nutrient standards, with around 30% to be supplied by school lunch (World Health Organization Recommendations on Diet, Nutrition and the Prevention of Chronic Disease 1990);

- sodium levels have been revised since the original report and are now based upon the current recommendations of The Scientific Advisory Committee on Nutrition. SACN (UK), 2003.

It is recognised that the consumption of a diet based on bread, cereals and other starchy foods, fruit and vegetables, and low amounts of fat, sugar and salty foods is a fundamental consideration in catering provision. The provision of food and drink, which meets these nutritional standards, is a key part of achieving a healthy dietary intake, but it is recognised that food provides considerably more than biological requirements. To perceive school food only in terms of nutrient delivery would be a missed opportunity for the development of social and life skills and for culinary richness.

Nutrient standards can be achieved in a variety of ways, which will involve consideration of menu planning (the composition of recipes used, the cooking and serving process), the product specification of individual food items, portion sizes and the frequency with which nutrient-dense foods are served during the school week.

Menu planning

To meet individual tastes the nutrient standards should be met by a choice of foods. Key points and menu-planning guidance is provided. Descriptors of foods and frequencies served are given as basic guidance for catering practice. It is emphasised that what is essential is the achievement of the nutrient standards. A flexible approach building on catering wisdom and experience, skills and local tastes is important in allowing a wide range of food and menu options to be available. It is important that good practice in menu design and food provision, which demonstrates the achievement of these standards, is shared amongst catering operatives. The Scottish Executive is commissioning the development of nutritional analysis software that will assist in the self-evaluation of nutrient standards.

Portion sizes

Portion size guidelines are necessary to assist caterers in planning lunches that meet nutrient standards for energy and other nutrients as well to satisfy young appetites. Hungry children are more likely to snack on high fat and sugar confectionery. Guidance on portion sizes is provided. In many cases schools will find that the portion sizes are substantially different from current practice. Larger portions of starchy food (bread, potatoes, pasta) and larger portions of fruit and vegetables will be required to meet the Scottish Nutrient Standards.

Product specifications

Product specifications are being developed to help plan menus to meet the Nutrient Standards and to raise the quality of manufactured products used in school lunches. Initial focus is being placed on fat and sodium content. They are being developed by the Food Standards Agency in Scotland. Consultation, particularly with the food industry, on the practicality, palatability and affordability of achieving such specifications will be an integral part of developing the specifications.

Drinking water

It is recognised that children need access to adequate amounts of fluids within the school day. Drinking water, which is free, fresh and chilled, should be provided with drinking cups or glasses within the dining room.

Food and drink choices

Promotion of appropriate food and drink choices is the responsibility of the whole school community. Within the dining room context there are specific issues that should be considered, including the following:

- awareness of appropriate choices (e.g. poster or other point of sale promotional materials, signposting and other visual cues);
- access to appropriate choices (e.g. counter positioning, easy access to promoted choices, less easy access to less favourable choices);
- availability of appropriate choices (e.g. ensuring sufficient provision of promoted items, especially such items as non-fried potatoes and salad);
- acceptability (e.g. promoted foods should taste good, be well cooked and attractively presented);
- affordability (e.g. appropriate pricing policy should be considered).

Special diets and allergies

Medically prescribed special dietary requirements should always be accommodated. Catering staff should be appropriately advised of the specific nature of the dietary requirement and children requiring special diets should be made known to the caterer. Diet guidance sheets should be provided by a State Registered Dietician in the form of detailed diet sheets or meal plans for the child concerned. This will indicate to the caterer the food choices that are suitable or should be excluded. The principle of variety and choice should apply equally where applicable to children on special diets as part of a wider child-centred approach to providing for these children.

Children and young people with special needs

Children and young people with special needs may have particular problems associated with eating. It is important that anyone involved in caring for children and young people with eating difficulties is trained to ensure that they can give the best and most appropriate assistance. These problems should not be a barrier to enjoyment and participation in meals and food choice or to learning about healthy eating.

Scottish nutrient standards for school lunches

These standards (Tables 1 and 2) are set for both the provision of food i.e. what the menu offers, and for the consumption of food i.e. what the child actually eats. The first of these, what the menu may offer, can be achieved by the caterer, but to influence the second will take a whole-school approach. Monitoring procedures will be set in place to monitor both the provision of food and the consumption of food by the child. The Scottish Nutrient Standards for School Lunches set out to ensure the provision of a meal that provides largely a third of a child's daily nutritional needs.

In Tables 1 and 2 the energy and nutrient requirements for children aged 5 to 18 years are presented as average values for males and females in three age groups. These guidelines provide figures for the recommended nutrient content of an average school lunch provided for children over one school week. In practical terms this is the amount of food provided, divided by the number of children eating it, averaged over a week. All the nutrient intakes in the tables are based on the average of the recommended intakes for boys and girls. The child's daily nutritional needs are expressed in terms of:

- dietary reference value (DRV) (or daily requirement);
- the reference nutrient intake (RNI) (the estimated amount of a nutrient that will meet the needs of most of the population);
- estimated average requirement (EAR) (in the tables EAR is used for energy to show the average requirement for energy for boys and girls).

It should be noted that current recommendations of energy intakes are based on children achieving a balance between energy intake and energy output allowing for growth and development. It is clear that children who are physically inactive will require less energy to meet physiological requirements and that excess energy will be a major contributor to the development of excess body weight. Both diet and physical activity are part of a holistic approach to maximising children's health.

To protect and to promote the health of children three nutrients are considered particularly significant. Calcium is important for bone growth. Iron is important for preventing anaemia, especially in secondary age schoolgirls. Folates are particularly important, again for secondary aged schoolgirls. It is recognised that some nutrients are supplied in high amounts in only a limited range of foods. The higher level of 40% of RNI for iron and folate has been adopted. In practice, levels have previously proved hard to achieve. However, because of the high health impact of a deficiency, efforts should be re-doubled to ensure adequate intakes.

It is recognised that these standards will take time to implement. Consultation undertaken by the Panel suggested that this will be more straightforward to implement in primary schools than in secondary and that schools will need time to incorporate changes into financial and development planning. It is expected that all schools will make rapid progress, but a final implementation date of December 2004 and December 2006 for primary and secondary respectively is expected.

Main recommendations

Education authorities and schools should have the Scottish Nutrient Standards for School Lunches in place in all special schools and primary schools by December 2004 and in all secondary schools by December 2006.

School meal should be monitored:

- as one of the curriculum priorities for 2003;
- as part of school inspections by Her Majesty's Inspection of Schools (HMI);
- as a commissioned task by HMI and specialist associate assessors 2004 to 2007.

Local authorities, who are the responsible agency for the provision of school meals, should incorporate their strategies with mainstream planning.

School meal facilities should not advertise nor promote food or drink with a high fat or high sugar content.

Table 1: Nutrient standards for school lunches for pupils in primary schools

			Unit	Infants 5-6 years	Junior 7-10 years
Energy	30% of EAR[1] Mean of girl and boy		MJ/Kcal	2,04 MJ 489 Kcal	2.33 MJ 557 Kcal
Fat	Not more than 35% food energy	Max	g	19	21.7
Saturated Fatty Acids	Not more than 11% food energy	Max	g	6	6.8
Carbohydrates	Not less than 50% food energy	Min	g	65,2	74.3
NME (non-milk extrinsic) Sugars[2]	Not more than 11% food energy	Max	g	14,3	16.3
Fibre/NSP (non-starch polysaccharides)[3]	Not less than 30% of calculated reference value	Min	g	3,9	4.5
Protein	Not less than 30% of RNI[4]	Min	g	5,9	8.5
Iron	Not less than 40 % of RNI	Min	mg	2,4	3.5
Calcium	Not less than 35 % of RNI	Min	mg	158	193
Vitamin A (retinol equivalents)	Not less than 30 % of RNI	Min	µg	150	150
Folate	Not less than 40 % of RNI	Min	µg	40	60
Vitamin C	Not less than 35 % of RNI	Min	mg	11	11
Sodium	Not more than 33% of SACN recommendation	Max	mg	393	655
Fruit and vegetables	1/3 of 5 portions per day		Portions	2	2

An extract from 'Hungry for success' Scottish Executive

1. Estimated average requirement
2. These are added sugars rather than the sugar that is integrally present in the food (e.g. table sugar, honey, sugar in fruit juice and soft drinks)
3. Here calculated as 8g per 1,000 kcal
4. Reference nutrient intake

Table 2: Nutrient standards school lunches for pupils in secondary schools

			Unit	All secondary 11-18 years
Energy	30% of EAR[1] Mean of boy and girl		MJ/Kcal	2.70 MJ 646 Kcal
Fat	Not more than 35% of food energy	Max	g	25.1
Saturated Fatty Acids	Not more than 11 % of food energy	Max	g	7.9
Carbohydrates	Not more than 50 % of food energy	Min	g	86.1
NME (non-milk extrinsic) Sugars[2]	Not more than 11 % of food energy	Max	g	18.0
Fibre/NSP (non-starch polysaccharides)[3]	Not less than 30% of food energy	Min	g	5.2
Protein	Not less than 30 % of RNI[4]	Min	g	13.3
Iron	Not less than 40 % of RNI	Min	mg	5.9
Calcium	Not less than 35 % of RNI	Min	mg	350
Vitamine A (retinol equivalents)	Not less than 30 % of RNI	Min	µg	185
Folate	Not less than 40 % of RNI	Min	µg	80
Vitamin C	Not less than 35 % of RNI	Min	mg	13
Sodium	Not more than 33 % of SACN recommendation	Max	mg	786
Fruit and vegetables	1/3 of 5 portions per day		Portions	2

An extract from 'Hungry for success' Scottish Executive

1. Estimated average requirement
2. These are added sugars rather than the sugar that is integrally present in food (e.g. table sugar, honey, sugar in fruit juice and soft drinks)
3. Here calculated as 8g per 1,000 kcal
4. Reference nutrient intake

References

Department of Health (DH). (1991). *Dietary Reference Values for Food Energy and Nutrients for the United Kingdom. Report of the Panel on Dietary Reference Values of the Committee on Medical Aspects of Food Policy.* Report on Health and Social Subjects. London: HMSO.

Caroline Walker Trust. (1992). *Nutritional Guidelines for School Meals. Report of an Expert Working Group.* London: Caroline Walker Trust.

Scottish Executive. (2003). *Hungry for Success. A Whole School Approach to School Meals in Scotland.* Edinburgh: The Stationery Office Bookshop. (See also website address, Appendix 3.)

Scientific Advisory Committee on Nutrition. (2003). *Salt and Health.* London: HMSO.

www.healthylivingscotland.gov.uk

How can school influence children's food choice and improve their diet?

Isabel LOUREIRO, Co-ordinator of Health Promotion and Protection, School of Public Health, Portugal.

The following are the extended highlights of a presentation by Isabel Loureiro, which sets the promotion of healthy eating in schools in the context of the research literature and policy development.

Eating: a health determinant

Appreciated as a vital factor and a source of pleasure and sharing, food is much more than nutrients: it has a special meaning for each person and group and it is part of one's identity. Eating is very dependent on personal factors and life circumstances.

Educating for eating well is one of the dimensions of the whole educational process, since nutrition is one of the most important health determinants, education should be seen in the context of wider public policies, inter-sectoral work and the empowerment of the communities and individuals.

It is estimated that more than a third of deaths due to cardiovascular disease in people under the age of 65 are attributable to diet[1] and that between 30 to 40 % of cancers can be attributed to dietary factors.[2] But eating can be salutogenic – either from a physical perspective or a mental one.[3] There are foods, such as fruit and vegetables, which can prevent some of these diseases as there are opportunities around eating which can structure the personality and reinforce the sense of coherence through affective bonds, family environment, coherence between messages and behaviours coming from adults.

According to the Institute of Public Health in Sweden the percentage of DALYs (disability-adjusted life-years) related to poor nutrition and physical inactivity is 9.7%.[4]

Portugal and Italy, accordingly to the WHO Health Report 2002[5] are the greatest consumers of fruit and vegetables in Europe. But Portugal also has the most sedentary population in the Region.

Group of countries	Vegetables (g/person per day)	Fruits (g/person per day	Fat (% of daily intake)
Italy and Portugal	243	196	30
Czech Republic, Hungary and Slovakia	239	180	35
Croatia, Slovenia and 'the former Yugoslav Republic of Macedonia'	241	155	37
Austria, Belgium and France	177	167	38
Baltic countries	198	176	41
Nordic countries	104	168	36
Azerbaijan, the Republic of Moldova and Ukraine	157	97	24
Kazakhstan, Kyrgyzstan and Uzbekistan	159	40	28

European Health Report 2002 (WHO, Regional Office for Europe, Copenhagen

Percentages of people in the EU countries who exercise insufficiently to benefit health (less than 3.5 hours per week), 1997

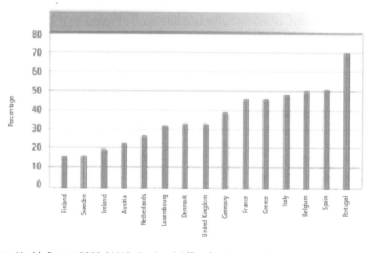

European Health Report 2002 (WHO, Regional Office for Europe, Copenhagen)

What the literature says about how to improve youth eating behaviour

According to a review on nutrition education research,[6] effective programmes to facilitate voluntary adoption of food and nutrition-related behaviours that are conducive to health and well-being use a combination of contemporary models of individual, social and environmental change. In young children, behavioural strategies included exposure to foods in a positive social context, modelling by peers and adults and appropriate use of rewards. For older children behavioural strategies included self-assessment, clarifying expectations and values, personal goal setting, and choosing among alternatives.

Critical ability seems an important variable to influence the ability to choose foods.[7] It has been associated with better food choices. Raising critical ability requires recognition of the rights of the child to express her/his points of view. Critical ability is raised through a systematic reflection on different situations, becoming aware of one's own thoughts and feelings, and confronting them with the knowledge acquired about the issue. It requires giving children the opportunity to learn, observe, judge, and choose by themselves.

It is important to have room for experiments or learning about nutrition can become 'dull' instead of pleasant.[8] To maintain interest on learning about foods, shifting from nutrients and focusing more on social dimension and personal living, can be a good learning strategy. As Levy-Strauss stated[9] "food is good to think".

An empowerment approach that includes enhancing personal control and self-efficacy proved to influence several health behaviours, including dietary choices. The whole person is a total and the values of each other determine behaviours in a systemic interconnection. For instance, people's own body image may have a strong influence on the eating habits, especially among adolescents, and this influence will interact with other health behaviours.

Reducing actual and perceived barriers to healthy choices remains an important public health objective. In a recent research about predicting adolescents' fruit and vegetable intake, Lytle and collaborators (2003), besides mentioning the importance of some predictors like subjective norms, knowledge, spirituality/religiosity, usual food choice and parenting style, concluded that the greater the barriers perceived, the fewer fruit and vegetables consumed.[10] The association between physical environmental-level factors and youth behaviour is clear in several studies.[11] Health promotion does not primarily address the individual: the main effort is to change and develop the physical and social environment.[12]

Philosophy and dimensions of Health Promoting Schools. Healthy eating: a human right

The network of Health Promoting Schools (HPS) finds its roots in the Ottawa Charter (WHO, 1986). Many values and practices were recognised as crucial for the development of health for all, such as participation, equity and empowerment. The Charter outlines a comprehensive strategy for health promotion through five interactive ways:

- building healthy public policy;
- creating supportive environments;
- strengthening community action;
- developing personal skills;
- reorientating health services;
- healthy public policy.

The HPS also fulfils the intention of the Convention on the Rights of the Child. In Article 12 No. 1, it is written:

> "States Parties shall assure to the child who is capable of forming his or her own views the right to express those views freely in all matters affecting the child, the views of the child being given due weight in accordance with the age and maturity of the child".

Article 13 No. 1 and article 24 No. 2 of the Convention are also supportive of the approach of health promotion in schools. Strategies for developing schools into health promoting settings put special emphasis on the following aspects:

- working for empowerment of students, teachers, other school staff, parents and other members of the community;
- investing in social capital (creating and reinforcing local networks, optimising local resources, increasing participation and family co-operation, sharing experiences and responsibilities);
- improving school organisational dimension for an holistic and comprehensive approach to health promotion through:
  - developing the ability to make a health diagnosis, select priorities and make a relevant plan of action;
  - integrating health issues into the curriculum;
  - using participative pedagogical methodologies;

- investing in the improvement of a healthy environment;
- building partnerships, mainly between the health and educational sectors and municipalities;
- advocating relevant policies at all levels;
- respecting the psychological and intellectual child development on choosing the messages and the methods of communication.

What makes sense on raising children (paternalism/empowerment)

Any intervention in a specific field, like nutrition, cannot be only focused on foods since eating behaviour also reflects how people control their instincts, care about themselves or how available they are for sharing with others. The way people eat shows how they relate with others, how much time and importance they give to it, what kind of cultural background they have, what their economic situation is. At home parents give messages to their children through the investment they put into mealtimes, including their ability to organise and plan the meal. It is also possible that they look for healthy alternatives in the short time they may have.

The short time to prepare foods should be taken into account not only by the industry but also by educators. Facilitating the acquisition of competencies of choice and preparation of quick meals is included in the learning objectives of nutrition education.

The HPS approach of improving eating behaviours is focused on enhancing health, besides reducing risk. The expected outcomes usually are to get specific behaviours and to improve the ability to make healthy choices; but an overall attitude towards the self as well as the knowledge and motivation to choose a healthy behaviour is required. Physical activity cannot be disregarded when looking for a body balance. As comprehensive health education, several behaviours are often targeted such as physical activity or smoking. Keeping them depends on a true personal will.

Empowerment in health promotion is imperative. According to Antonovsky, central to the concept of salutogenesis is the sense of coherence. For the process of raising children, the sense of coherence approach seems appropriate when we think about the importance of the sense of meaningfulness (motivational component), the sense of comprehensibility (cognitive processing of stimuli), and the sense of manageability (cognitive emotional processing) - the three components of this model.[13]

School menus should take into account pupils' preferences, eating habits and values related to foods and meals. Nutrition education should start from there to be meaningful. Participation in decision-making has to be socially recognised as relevant. "Individuals' values form an important part of the motivation system".[14]

Coherence between messages, adult behaviour and the food offered, at least in school and at home, contribute to consistency; within the school it is crucial that messages learnt in the classroom match what and how foods are presented at the buffet and /or canteen. For the component of manageability, nutrition problems and socio-economic characteristics of the community, along with the knowledge about nutrient and calorific needs, are basic information to understand if manageability is possible. Capacity building is important to make students feel in control, like getting competencies for making a recipe, taking decisions about what foods should be acquired for the buffet or having good manners at the table. Teachers and school have to find ways to get pupils interested in choosing healthy foods, learning by doing and allowing their creativity as well as testing their self-efficacy on preparing snacks and meals. The belief that resources are available depends on one's own resources and others' resources or belief on a higher power that can assist in successfully dealing with difficulties.

One of the main reasons teachers give for not making the canteen or the buffet a context for nutrition education (giving opportunities to the students for developing competencies of healthy choices, preparation of snacks and cooking foods) is the lack of human resources and budget to acquire the adequate equipment and make some physical changes in the environment. In any case, many things have been done even with these difficulties.

National and local policies are also needed to assure the sense of manageability. A national policy to regulate the requirements about the safety of the environment, specifically on production and manipulation of foods, regulations about nutrition at schools, with local accountability, should be compulsory. Publicity regulation is another responsibility for the government. With an empowerment approach, decision-taking is assumed at all levels and the capacity of social organisation increases by growing autonomy, self-efficacy and networking. According to the level of empowerment, the quality of democracy and civic participation determine, by level of social capital, a potential to produce positive changes.

A description of a pilot project in Portugal, which is based on the preceding models was then elucidated, the text of this appears in the proceedings of the forum.

Reference Notes

1. European Heart Network (1998) – Food, nutrition, and cardiovascular disease prevention in Europe.

   European Heart Network, Brussels. In: Societé Française de Santé Publique (2000) – Health and Human nutrition: element for European action. Présidence française de l'Union Européenne, Ministère de l'Emploi et de la Solidarité de la République Française. Collection Santé & Societé n° 10.

2. Doll, R; Peto, R. (1981) – The cause of cancer: quantitative estimates of avoidable risks of cancer in the United States today. J Natl Cancer Ins, 66: 1191-1308. In: Societé Française de Santé Publique (2000) – Health and Human nutrition: element for European action. Présidence française de l'Union Européenne, Ministère de l'Emploi et de la Solidarité de la République Française. Collection Santé & Societé n° 10.

3. Antonovsky, A. (1996) – The salutogenic model as a theory to guide health promotion. Health Promotion International, 11: 11-18.

4. Referred in the European Health Report 2002 of WHO.

5. WHO (2002) – The European Health Report 2002. Copenhagen, WHO, Regional Office for Europe.

6. A review of nutrition education research was accomplished by Isobel Contento taking into account 217 nutrition education intervention studies. Contento, I. (1996) – The effectiveness of nutrition education and implications for nutrition education policy: programs, and research: a review of research. Society for nutrition Education, 27: (6) p.277-421.

7. Loureiro, I. (1994) – Indução de práticas alimentares saudáveis nos primeiros anos de escolaridade. Ph.D. thesis. Lisboa. Universidade Nova de Lisboa. Unpublished.

8. From article kindly provided by Jette Benn, in 1997 "Nutrition education in question: a critical educational approach to nutrition education in schools". The Royal Danish School of Educational Studies, Department of Biology, Geography and Home Economics, Copenhagen.

9. Benn in her work about "Nutrition education in question: a critical educational approach to nutrition education in schools" (1997) mentions this expression by Levy-Strauss.

10. Lytle, L.A. (2003) – Predicting adolescents' intake of fruit and vegetables. J Nutr Educ Behav. 2003; 35: 170-178.

11. Story M. et al (1996) – Availability of foods in high schools: is there cause for concern? J Am Diet Assoc 1996; 96: 123-126.

12. Grossmann, R.; Scala, K.C. (1996) – Health promotion and organizational development: developing settings for health. Vienna, WHO, Regional Office for Europe, Health Promotion Unit, Lifestyles and Health Department.

13. Antonovsky, A. (1979). 'Health, stress and coping: new perspective on mental and physical wellbeing'. San Francisco, CA., Jossey-Bass.

14. Tones, K. (2003) – Health promotion, health education, and the public health In: Public Health. In: Detels, R. et al (2002) - Oxford textbook of Public Health: the methods of Public Health. Oxford, Oxford University Press. p.p. 829-863.

15. Lee, R.J.; Freedman, A.M. (1984) – Consultation skills Alexandria, VA.

16. International Obesity Task Force (WHO Nutrition Unit).

Discussion: Healthy eating in schools

At the end of the presentations in session one there was an opportunity to raise questions arising from the contributions as well as to respond to specific questions raised by the facilitator of the session Jeltje Snel.

The subject of supervision of meals was raised.........

Meta Schuster (Sweden). How do you work to get teachers in the dining room?

Gillian Kynoch (Scotland) stated that if the food and environment are good enough for the teachers, it should be good enough for the pupils. The place where the teachers are eating should be used as a benchmark.

Tony Apicella (England). As a former headteacher, it should be recognised that teachers may want space from the young people at lunchtime. We should remember that other staff such as learning support assistants have a role to play.

Richard Coudyser (France). To begin with, teachers in France were present in the dining room, but this is disappearing. If teachers volunteer to supervise they may be paid from the municipal budget.

On the subject of provision, uptake and choice of meals........

Finnish Delegate. In Finland meals are provided free of charge to all pupils but you cannot make the young people eat it – school culture and other factors define the uptake in our country.

Beeltje Liefers (Netherlands). As a caterer I believe you can start to create a balance – a free choice is necessary.

Ferdy Naafs (Netherlands). Our Association consulted members on whether schools should offer meals or not in all schools.

Ines Heindl (Germany). Parents took over food provision in some schools in Westphalia – this started on a voluntary basis.

On the subject of fruit and snacks.........

Doris Kuhness (Austria). Pupils can create their own healthy snacks, we need to involve the students.

Carmen Perez Rodrigo (Spain). Due to an intervention in parts of Spain, supported by the European Commission, they now have a fruit break in some schools.

Anniken Owren Aarum (Norway). Our school fruit programme has had an impact on intake but we have learned that we need to involve parents and kindergartens more.

Rachel Thom (England). In some counties in England all children are now receiving free fruit and it is starting to increase parental interest and involvement.

Bent Mikkelsen (Denmark). One important partner we sometimes miss are the growers and suppliers – we need to make fruit easier to eat by helping them to develop more convenient products.

And finally........

Ines Heindl. When we come up with recommendations we have to start with people's cultural background.

Healthy eating in the traditional school meals system. The role of the private food service operator

Richard Coudyser, Director General, Sodexho, France

Richard Coudyser of Sodexho, the largest private company involved in school meals production in Europe, explained the approach of his company and the partnership role of the private food service operator in the future. These are the extended highlights of his presentation.

Introduction

Session No. 2 is concerned with how to provide healthy food in schools. A number of key issues were raised in the introduction to the session. From a catering company's standpoint four main ideas should be underlined:

First, promoting healthy eating in schools necessitates the existence of high-quality, efficient school meals services. For private catering operators this translates into stricter contractual requirements to:

- offer balanced, healthy menus;
- create conditions conducive to the dissemination of good eating habits;
- give pupils the freedom to make healthy food choices;
- involve pupils in composing their meals once they are of an age to do so.

Second, the observation that responsibility for healthy meal provision has gradually shifted from the parents to the school. In other words, the school canteen is now subject not only to an obligation of means, but also to an obligation of results and is constantly being judged by parents, who have become more demanding.

Third, there is a cultural dimension peculiar to each country. Eating habits, the importance attached to lunch hour and attitudes towards private companies delivering public services vary from one country to another. It is for this reason that the basic model of school meals provision differs in northern Europe, the United Kingdom and France.

Fourth, promoting healthy eating in schools largely depends on the public-private partnership's ability to delimit clearly the fields of competence of the client public authority and the private operator, to listen to each other and to work together in pursuit of shared objectives.

However, this is an area where debate may be influenced by ideology. In France, but doubtless also in other European countries, some people are extremely wary of private operators. They believe that in a private company the profit imperative is, by nature, antithetical to satisfaction of a public service need, such as provision of school meals. We are all familiar with received ideas along the lines that the profit motive prevents private operators from taking innovative steps, which might reduce their margin, or that responsibility for school meals should continue to lie with the public authorities and private operators should confine themselves to meal production and delivery.

Although such hackneyed opinions die hard, it must nonetheless be acknowledged that there are intrinsic advantages to privatising school meals. A private company can harness its financing capacity to the public authority's needs. It is on this very principle that the system of delegating public services as we know it in France is based. A private firm is often more responsive and flexible than its public counterpart. It is also capable of innovating, and developing healthy school meals service concepts.

Our aim is to answer the question: What should be the private food service operator's role in providing healthy food in the traditional school meals system? Sodexho is the world and European leader in the catering services market. It is present in 74 countries on almost 25,000 sites, which has enabled it to develop expert know-how in this field of activity, of which school meals are one aspect.

How does Sodexho, as a private food services provider, respond to the challenges of changing eating patterns and concerns about young people's health both in designing its menus and in the field of nutrition education? Sodexho's objective is to ensure that the children's nutritional requirements are met, and we shall look at the results of a newly released survey on healthy eating, conducted by the Sodexho Research Institute into the Quality of Daily Life in 2002 among UK schoolchildren and their parents.

Sodexho's commitments regarding menu design and taste and nutrition education

School meals are pivotal to the issue of the food-products offer and nutrition education and the school canteen constitutes an alternative place of learning, different from the home and the classroom. Although it is true that of the 21 meals eaten per week only four or five are taken at school, the canteen may nonetheless be an ideal place to educate children's taste buds and teach them to differentiate what they eat. Unlike nutrition education in the classroom, forming part of the school curriculum, the canteen offers immediate opportunities for 'practical work'. In addition, on returning home, children can raise their parents' awareness of what in practice constitutes a healthy, balanced diet.

From the point of view of promoting healthy eating, the school canteen can fulfil two functions:

- it can directly influence food intake by offering children balanced menus and food products;
- it can facilitate nutrition education by enabling children to see for themselves how their meals balance.

Sodhexo has decided to treat these two functions as two priority objectives. We accordingly pay special attention to the design of the menus we offer children. We also help to train municipal catering staff in the pedagogic aspects of nutrition education and taste education.

Answering the nutritional needs of those partaking of our meals (children, adolescents, young adults) is a pillar of Sodexho's quality policy. To that end, we focus on three main objectives:

- taking the public health dimension into account: 'learning to eat well for future health' is our credo;
- contributing to nutrition education and taste education;
- integrating the concept of eating for pleasure in menu design.

These objectives are reflected in our commitments regarding menu design:

- compliance with the standards and regulations in force and monitoring of any changes in them;
- appraising user satisfaction on a daily basis for each menu choice in each school;
- affording school access to research results and advice provided by our panel of scientific advisers on nutrition;
- encouraging consumption of fruit and vegetables by supplying ripe produce;
- encouraging consumption of complex carbohydrates by giving bread a higher profile and offering original legume-based recipes;
- encouraging consumption of fish, by including it more often on our menus (offering three fish choices over a two-week period).

To ensure eating is also a pleasurable experience, we have set ourselves specific criteria regarding menu design:

- use of seasonal dishes and products;
- serving harmonised meals, taking account of food colour, texture and combinations;
- direct appraisal of pupils' satisfaction:
  - ⇨ each school has a 'tasting club': we bring together 12 children five times a year to test and approve new dishes and recipes which will be included on the menu over the following weeks;
  - ⇨ a measurer which we call 'C' mon goût': we measure the quantities actually consumed for each dish, each day in each school;
- the school managing body's menu committee, which identifies recipes and products to be improved;
- seeking and creating new recipes with four well-known French chefs: Michel Bras, Jean-Michel Lorain, Olivier Roellinger and Jacques Chilbois.

One of the key focuses of this innovative approach is knowledge, cooking and seasoning of green vegetables.

How does Sodexho take health into account in its menus?

- by ensuring compliance with the circular of 25/06/2001 on the composition of school meals and food safety;
- by encouraging consumption of fruit, vegetables, fish and complex carbohydrates;
- by providing information and advice through our panel of scientific experts on nutrition;
- by relying on a team of dieticians, who verify on a day-to-day basis that the meals we serve are good for the well-being of those who eat them.

Sodexho has set itself the task of helping to make children receptive to good eating practices and participating in educating their taste buds. The success of this learning experience depends on a range of simple measures, involving in-class teaching, which must be followed up in the school canteen. On request, Sodexho can mobilise its nutrition expertise, culinary know-how and dieticians. This awareness-raising exercise must enable children to acquire the right habits. Nor are parents forgotten, since we do everything we can to encourage children to share their new knowledge with other family members.

We have developed specific schemes for what we call the 'Small-but-big kids' (children aged three to seven) and the 'Stars' (those aged seven to 12).

Since 1990 Sodexho's UK subsidiary has been publishing a school meals survey, conducted on a regular basis by the Sodexho research services. This survey is the most significant in quantitative and qualitative terms, and also the most ambitious, of the entire catering services industry. The 2002 survey was the seventh of its kind.

One of the merits of the 2002 report is that it comes 18 months after the national authorities introduced nutritional standards for lunches served in school canteens in England. For the 2002 survey a representative sample of 1,608 children aged five to 16 was interviewed, as well as 1,413 parents. The results indicated the following:

- the frequency of eating chips has been falling regularly nationwide since 1994. From three times per week in 1994 it had decreased to 2.25 times per week in 2002;

- 68% of the children interviewed said that their diet was very or quite healthy. This was 6% lower than in 2000;

- 60% of parents thought the meals served by their child's school were very or quite healthy;

- the top three reasons why children said their diet was healthy were, by order of importance, eating lots of fruit (50%), eating lots of vegetables (44%) and eating a balanced diet (20%). However, the survey results showed that overall consumption of fruit and vegetables by children was in fact very low;

- 45% of children who said their diet was unhealthy attributed this to eating too many sweets and chocolates. 34% said it was due to eating junk or fast food, whereas 30% put it down to eating too many chips;

- 37% of the children interviewed would be ready to choose healthy foods at school if the menu choices were more varied. 18% said the taste of healthy food options at school must be improved before they would choose them;

- on average, fruit was eaten 3.88 times a week, compared with 3.79 times for vegetables. However, these frequencies rose to 4.12 and 3.89 respectively where the school had a food advisory committee;

- more schools were dealing with healthy eating issues. In 2002, 68% of the children interviewed said these matters had been addressed during the school year, compared with 60% in 2000. Where the school had a food group, 84% of the children said healthy eating was discussed in class;

- 85% of parents considered it important or very important that schools raise their children's awareness about a good, balanced diet. 67% of parents said the principles taught at school had had a visible or fairly visible impact on children's attitudes at home, whereas the 2000 figure was 62%;

- 47% of children said their school encouraged healthy eating, but this rose to 67% where there was a school food advisory committee. The survey therefore showed the proven success of food groups and committees, while highlighting the failure of policies pursued by schools without such bodies;

- of 7 million schoolchildren in the UK, only 790,000 are aware of the existence of food groups and committees, and less than 253,000 take part in them or are indirectly involved;

- in conclusion, it can be said that UK children do know what a healthy diet is, but this does not mean that their eating behaviour follows the relevant criteria.

Conclusion

a. The fact that governments - whether the French Government with its circular on school meals composition of 25 June 2001 or the UK Government with the nutritional standards for school lunches introduced in April 2001 - deemed it necessary to lay down rules testifies to the lack of nutritional balance previously observed in school meals.

Although it is true that only four or five meals per week are taken at school, we believe that the school canteen can be an excellent place to educate children's taste buds and teach them about nutrition. Nor does this situation mean that the school caterer is not obliged to ensure that all children taking school meals, whether attending state or private schools, are offered menus providing a perfectly balanced diet.

b. The private catering services operator cannot be made a scapegoat for the nutritional imbalances observed in some menus proposed in schools. In France, for example, the fact that responsibility for managing school canteens is shared among many different operators can mean that catering companies are marginalised (private catering firms are all but absent from state secondary schools) and, more often than not, relegated to the role of mere production and delivery of meals (in state nursery and primary schools the relationship between the client municipal authority and the catering sub-contractor more closely resembles a top-down chain of command than a genuine partnership).

c. To meet the challenges of a varied, healthy diet and nutrition education, Sodexho has made innovation a key feature of its approach. This is why the menu choices we offer children incorporate a public-health dimension (learning to eat properly for future health), without disregarding the need for a constant effort to improve tastes and flavours, which help to make mealtimes a pleasurable experience. Moreover, to remain competitive vis-à-vis our rivals, we have chosen to focus on what our users have to say. It was for this reason that we conducted our first major survey of UK schoolchildren in 1994. This is also what we seek to do day-after-day in each school through measures such as the taste clubs and use of the *'C' mon goût'* measurer.

d. At a European level Sodexho wishes to help enhance knowledge of what constitutes a healthy, balanced diet for children. It also seeks to encourage the implementation of a global, multidisciplinary approach in such matters. It is our view that statistical and scientific knowledge of school meals is still too fragmented and embryonic. In addition, many parties are involved in promoting healthy eating in schools - teachers, paediatricians, politicians, parents, etc. However, their action more often than not lacks co-ordination because there is no global, multidisciplinary approach.

With these issues in mind, Sodexho recently launched a European healthy eating programme concerning the fifteen EU member states plus Norway, Poland and Slovakia. This programme is being implemented in partnership with four major education sector players:

- the European Association of Paediatricians;
- the European Trade Union Committee for Education (ETUCE), which brings together 81 teachers' unions;
- the European Parents' Association (EPA), which represents 100 million parents;
- a European network of elected representatives in local government.

The results of this huge survey will be made public in February 2004 in connection with a first European conference on healthy eating, aimed at initiating a public debate and fostering a multi disciplinary approach, involving all those participating in school life. This event will seek to define joint objectives for all the groups of operators concerned by healthy eating in schools. These objectives will then be adapted to the individual countries, and a monitoring process will be implemented to gauge the effectiveness of the measures taken.

School fruit programmes as a short cut to promoting healthy eating in schools – The Norwegian experience

Anniken OWREN AARUM, Directorate for Health and Social Affairs, Norway

This paper sets out the important lessons learned, including cost and quality factors, in introducing a school fruit programme in primary and lower secondary school stages in Norway.

Introduction

A national survey conducted in 1993 in Norway, found that the average fruit consumption among 13-year-olds was only about two portions a day. The Norwegian Directorate for Health and Social Affairs recommends 'at least five a day'. In Norway, school lunch for most children consists of open-faced sandwiches brought from home, and few students tend to bring fruit or vegetables as part of their lunch-packs. In 1996 a decision was taken to launch a pilot test of a school subscription scheme, for fruit and vegetables in primary and lower secondary schools (called 'School Fruit'), like the school milk subscription scheme. The programme has now been introduced in 18 of Norway's 19 counties. This presentation will outline the experiences we have gained from this programme.

Physical availability, educational, financial and normative measures for increasing participation

The Schools Fruit programme is a public–private partnership, and it is being implemented in co-operation between the Norwegian Fruit and Vegetables Marketing Board and the Directorate for Health and Social Affairs, the county health authorities and private, local wholesale distributors. For Norwegian Kroner 2.50 (€0.30) a day, each participating pupil receives an apple, a pear, carrot, clementine, banana or other fruit at lunch. A comprehensive information and marketing campaign has been conducted targeting school administrators and staff, pupils and their parents, wholesalers and health service personnel. Great emphasis has also been placed on obtaining funding and legislation to promote school and pupil participation. In the past four years the programme has been granted €1.25 million in subsidies through a collective agricultural agreement between Norway's farmers and the agricultural authorities. The schools themselves determine whether to offer fruit, vegetables or other food. The Directorate has drawn up official guidelines for school meals advising schools to offer fruit and vegetables as a supplement to milk and sandwiches. Regulations concerning the school environment recommend that these guidelines be observed. The challenge facing us is to exploit more effectively the opportunities that exist within the present framework in order to increase school participation.

Experience to date

Approximately 56,000 pupils in 830 schools participated in the programme in the spring of 2003. On average, about 35% of the pupils from schools that are participating in the programme subscribe to the school fruit scheme. This means about 28% of Norway's primary and lower secondary schools. The goal is that all schools should introduce a fruit and vegetable subscription scheme.

The University of Oslo has investigated the effect of the school fruit programme on the consumption of fruit and vegetables in an intervention study, 'Fruit and vegetables in the 6th form', with the objective of developing effective strategies for promoting sufficient intake of fruit and vegetables. The study was conducted among 12-year-old pupils in 38 primary schools. At ten of the intervention schools, the pupils were served fruit and vegetables free of charge during one year. The intervention components were a classroom curriculum in home economics that included Internet-based learning, fruit and vegetables made available at school through the school fruit programme, and a family component with information both at home and at school. Preliminary results show that participation in the school fruit subscription scheme yielded an increase in consumption of 0.4 portions/day. Targeted instruction alone did not influence consumption. Among the pupils who had access to free fruit and vegetables, consumption increased by 0.7 portions/day.

Data from a school meal survey in 2000 indicates that establishing a school fruit programme also prompts more pupils to bring fruit and vegetables from home. The results of market surveys show that 80% of all parents would like the schools to offer subscription schemes for fruit and vegetables (SSB 2001), but no parents are willing to pay more than the current price. Half of the parents would like the price to be lower than at present or free of charge (2003). Process evaluation data show that insufficient time for administration, a lack of cool-storage facilities, and scepticism about parental payment because not all pupils can participate are the most important arguments against the school fruit programme at schools that are not participating in the scheme.

Challenges ahead

In order to increase participation in the programme by schools and pupils, variation and top quality products must be ensured throughout the country, new products that are ready to be served must be developed, the schools' administration of the programme must be simplified, and communication with schools, parents and local authorities must be improved.

It is a dilemma that some pupils probably do not participate because of the price. The frequency and time of payment may influence participation. The programme could conceivably increase rather than reduce social health disparities related to fruit and vegetable consumption. For this reason the White Paper on public health points out the need to document the effect of the subscription price on the intake of fruit and vegetables among children and adolescents.

Although much remains to be done before all schools in Norway have established school fruit programmes or similar schemes, we see that it is possible to increase participation by both schools and pupils substantially through various measures now being implemented.

In conclusion, it is suggested that the following actions increase success:

• employ a range of different measures (normative, educational, material);

• create an open dialogue with suppliers;

• draw up a contract specifying quality and variation;

• circulate useful experience and examples of organisation among schools

• offer practical help to schools;

• establish regular contact persons at the schools;

• use the media and local collaborating partners in information activities

• be patient.

The home-made lunchbox – has it got a future?

Doris KUHNESS, Manager, Program 'Healthy school', Styria vitalis, Austria

This paper makes the case for the lunchbox or packed lunch having the potential to provide a healthy school lunch

With young people we can find three main problems in regard to their health. These are smoking, irregular diet and lack of exercise. Besides eating food with essential nutrients, eating regularly is an indicator of healthy nourishment. On the basis of that we must say that 23% of the 11–15 year old girls have insufficient and 25% have problematic eating habits.

A balanced diet is very important for the development of children and young people. They normally do not consider the health aspects of nourishment. Apart from the satisfaction of their needs, other factors play important roles: fast food is fun, eating and drinking depend on contemporary trends. In addition to this the proportion of overweight children in the lower classes is clearly higher than in the upper classes. These differences indicate different eating habits in various social strata. Apart from the irregular eating habits, the lack of exercise has a negative influence on the BMI (Body Mass Index) and consequently on the health of young people.

Extensive educational and information activities as well as programmes aimed at providing knowledge about prevention of bad nutritional habits have shown that knowing more about healthy nourishment does not really lead to more sensible eating habits of young people. For there is still a big discrepancy between what young people like to eat on the one hand and modern recommendations for healthy food on the other.

The most popular school lunch usually still includes a sausage sandwich and lemonade, the healthiest, however, should consist of coarse wholemeal bread, milk and fruit.

This indicates clearly that the strategies we have adopted so far, such as comprehensive information and the attempts to make a healthy school lunch more attractive in regard to being enjoyed and having a favourable image, have only had modest results.

If we realise that, how can the school together with the parents proceed in an innovative way in order to improve the health of young people through a change of nutritional habits? School is not only a place where knowledge is provided but it also has considerable influence on the health of pupils and teachers. Experience with the concept of Health Promoting Schools shows that lasting improvements can be achieved if education at schools and health projects are based on the principles of health promotion:

- to organise schools as a health promoting environment: encourage the participation of those who are affected in the process of change (settings approach);
- promote the individual competences and abilities of the pupils to lead healthy lives (empowerment);
- establish a network of the school with partners in the region;
- develop health measures that take into consideration physical, psychological and social aspects;
- encourage the communication and co-operation between teachers, parents and pupils.

A school project 'Design your snack' was set up to explore the ideas of pupils on the topic of lunchboxes and to determine if the lunchbox under certain conditions can contribute towards healthy nutritional habits. The aims of the project were:

- activation for a healthier school lunch;
- to improve the quality of the snacks sold in school;
- to increase the participation of pupils.

The target group were pupils aged 11 to 15. Pupils created their own healthy snacks and developed the system for merchandising (packing and selling).

The outcomes were better quality snacks offered at school buffets and pupils becoming actively involved in the improvement in quality of the lunchboxes. In addition 45% of the parents in the healthy schools made changes to their eating habits. These included an increase in the consumption of potatoes, rice, vegetables and wholemeal bread and a reduction in meat consumption. Parents also demonstrated an increase in knowledge and children were buying less sweets and sweet drinks and drinking more water.

It is concluded that the home-made lunchbox or packed lunch provides an opportunity for parents to reflect on and change their nutrition behaviour. Further details of the work referred to in these projects can be seen at www.daisy.at and at www.styriavitalis.at

Discussion: How to provide healthy food in schools

After the presentations, the facilitator Vivian Rasmussen gave an opportunity to delegates who wished to ask the presenters questions or to comment on the provision of healthy food in schools.

On the subjects of policy and accountability.......

Aileen Robertson (WHO). With reference to the paper from Norway on school fruit programmes, delegates should know that WHO are promoting fruit and vegetables in a new joint initiative with FAO. In the 'Food and Nutrition Action Plan', governments will be assessed in terms of what they are doing to promote healthy eating.

On the subject of food, the environment and sustainability.......

Delegate from Hamburg, (Germany). It is important to use organic food in school healthy eating programmes.

Anniken Owren Aarum, (Norway). Organic products are included in the Norwegian scheme.

Rachel Thom (England) referred to a list of projects in England, which were making links between food production and the land, such as 'growing schools' and 'learning through landscapes'. (see Appendix 3).

Ian Young (Rapporteur) supported this point and added the names of 'Grounds for Learning' and 'Eco-schools', which include the link between food production and the environment. (see Appendix 3).

Stefka Petrova (Bulgaria) referred to the importance of work in schools, which helped the understanding of food production in relation to the land. She explained that in Bulgaria they had developed a book of traditional Bulgarian recipes to encourage healthy eating.

Carmen Perez Rodrigo (Spain) mentioned the initiative in Spain, which encourages school farms as integral to learning about food and its production.

Mark Karaczun (England) asked the question what is a school meal? He described an interesting project in the Veneto in Italy, where local, organic food is sourced for schools. Many parents were initially sceptical about giving more vegetables to their children but gradually they accepted the argument that it was beneficial to the health of their children. He also referred to the East Anglia food link website www.eafl.org.uk which links food production, health and sustainable development in that part of England. (see Appendix 3).

On the subject of lunchboxes from a country with colder winters........

Kaija Hartiala (Finland) referring to the paper on the home-made lunchbox, stated that 95% of children in Finland had a hot meal provided every day free of charge. She suggested that the lunchbox was not a good option as the children need a hot meal.

Ian Young (Rapporteur) suggested the need to share information on website addresses and that this could perhaps be incorporated into the report.

School food policy: Linking with the Netherlands healthy schools action programme

Goof BUIJS, Netherlands Institute for Health Promotion and Disease Prevention.

Goof Buijs describes how we should grasp the opportunity of the higher political profile of healthy eating by involving schools in planning the solutions rather than telling them what needs to be done.

Introduction

There are many good reasons to pay attention to health and the promotion of a healthy lifestyle for young people in Europe. By this we mean addressing risk behaviours such as drinking of alcohol, smoking, unhealthy eating, lack of physical activity. Taking risks when you are young is part of the process of growing up. Young people need to learn to get these risks within acceptable boundaries and also how to keep these boundaries acceptable. Disease prevention and health promotion are an important tool in this learning process.

When you think of youth, you think of schools. Schools are a suitable setting to reach young people with health promotion. This is preferably done through an integral approach, which implies more than just teaching health education in the classroom. Recently in the Netherlands the Co-ordinated School Health Programme Model has been introduced.

In the national action programme on health promoting schools the school itself has been given the central position. What are the needs and demands from a school in the area of health, and how can we organise support for schools? Too many projects have been presented to the school, which they have not asked for. Collaboration on local, regional and national level is crucial.

Nutrition is one of the key issues in school health promotion. In this paper, I will describe the current developments in the Netherlands in the area of health promoting schools. A new policy paper on prevention puts health promoting schools in a central place. I will demonstrate how healthy eating can be linked with the demand-oriented approach. There is a growing political interest in the issue of overweight. This offers sudden new opportunities for school food policy as one of the key settings to prevent overweight among schoolchildren. European collaboration in this area, which has been demonstrated over the past decade by the development of the spiral curriculum of nutrition education, can provide stimulating and new thinking in this area.

Dutch Action Programme

Health promotion in schools is fragmented and hardly ever addresses the needs of a specific school and its pupils and staff. In 2002 the Netherlands action programme on promoting health in schools was presented. The programme consists of a coherent vision on the future development of health promoting schools in the Netherlands. The three main goals of the programme are:

1. to improve collaboration between organisations on local, regional and national level:
- exchanging initiatives, instruments and experiences;
- developing new initiatives;
- linking with youth policy;
- on the political and working agendas.

2. to improve information and transfer of knowledge
- marketing the health promoting school concept;
- setting a national support centre;
- running a website on health promoting schools;
- masterclass health promoting schools.

3. to improve the quality of interventions for health promoting schools:
- basic curriculum on health education from four to 16 years;
- research on effectiveness of interventions;
- standardisation of questionnaires, protocols, etc.

The collaboration between the health and the education sector has been given priority in this programme.

Growing impact

Ever since the action programme was launched, there is a growing impact of and shared interest in the issue of health promoting schools. I will mention four important developments:

1. In Autumn 2003 the Dutch Government published the national policy paper on Prevention. In this document investment in the health of young people has been given a priority. Schools have been identified as the most important setting for reaching young people. The policy paper offers new opportunities for getting health promoting schools on the political agenda.

2. The thirty large cities in the Netherlands are developing the large city policy for the period 2005-2009; for the first time a paragraph on health will be included, mainly on reducing inequalities in health. In this policy paper health promoting schools has been made one of its spearheads. Municipalities are becoming more and more aware of their role in promoting the health of their citizens.

3. Supervised by the Ministry of Health, eight national institutes are working together on a joint working plan 2004 health promoting schools. These institutes work mostly on a single health issue (such as nutrition, smoking and safety) and are funded by the ministry. This collaboration is in line with the national action programme on health promoting schools and can be regarded as a unique step forward in a more co-ordinated approach.

4. Local authorities are responsible for their own health policy, the 40 regional services carry out this policy. They play a key role in supporting schools in the area of health. A number of regional innovative projects help to set the agenda for health promoting schools nationally. One example is the Schoolbeat Project (www.schoolslag.nl) in Maastricht Region: an innovative regional approach to health promotion and preventative care in schools. Schoolbeat aims to reduce risk behaviour in youth (4 to 19 years) over a ten-year period. There is a focus on responding to needs and demands of individual schools and their communities.

I would like to refer to the Egmond Agenda, that was adopted at the European Conference on Health Promoting Schools: Education and Health in Partnership in the Netherlands in September 2002. This agenda provides a helpful tool for developing a national strategy where health and education can actually meet and work together.

The co-ordinated school health programme model

For a better understanding of school health promotion the American Co-ordinated School Health Programme Model (CSHP-model) has been introduced, first in the regional Schoolbeat project and next in the national action programme. The model is currently being tailored to the Dutch situation.

Each of the components of the model supports empowerment, involvement of pupils and parents, improvement in schools' health culture and incorporation of health promotion in the existing pupil care structure. The advantage of this comprehensive approach is that it enables schools to build upon existing health activities and projects. It offers a systematic way of developing school health activities in a way that has been proven the most effective and promising.

Quality care in schools

Most schools in general are initially not very interested in investing in health promotion, because they see it as extra work on an already overloaded agenda. Schools do not ask for more work, they ask for support to meet their needs. Health promotion has to make clear what the added value is to the core business of a school. I would like to refer to the experience in the United Kingdom with the Healthy Schools Scheme, which has demonstrated its impact on school improvement. It is essential to get a good and complete view on the needs and wishes of schools in the area of health. In the Netherlands a number of instruments have been developed and are now being implemented in Schoolbeat and other pilot projects. Each of the instruments help to clarify the demands from a school and to set priorities on dealing with health issues as a basis for a school plan.

A recent key for promoting health in schools is the linking with the pupil's care in schools. Schools currently experience many difficulties in acquiring adequate care for students with 'problems'. To ensure successful tailor-made school health promotion a chain-care approach is being constructed for linking school health promotion with individual pupil care. Top priority in schools nowadays is quality care: for us this offers the opportunity to introduce health promotion!

Linking with school food policy

One of the components of the Co-ordinated School Health Programme is the provision of school nutrition services. I will give you an example of how to link the issue of nutrition with each of the eight components of the CSHP Model.

1. Health education in the classroom
   Comprehensive nutrition programme based on the spiral curriculum for nutrition education from 4 to 16 years. Focusing on nutrition as a healthy lifestyle issue. Development of programmes that work should be given priority.

2. School nutrition services
   Offering a varied, affordable and healthy selection of meals, snacks and drinks. Creating an environment that enhances healthy eating behaviour. Pupils have better learning results when they are eating well.

3. Physical education (sports and exercise)
   Promoting a physical active life. Physical education is meant to help young people to acquire the necessary skills and to improve physical fitness. It also enhances mental, social and emotional skills. And it is one of the main influences on the prevention of weight gain.

4. School health services
   Focusing on adequate monitoring, guidance and reference of pupils with problems in the area of nutrition. This can be both overweight and underweight, lack of healthy diet, etc.

5. School counselling, psychological and social services
   Guidance and support focusing on the cognitive, emotional, behavioural and social needs of pupils and its social environment. Its goal is to prevent problems and to stimulate a healthy mental development.

6. Healthy school environment
   A safe, clean and well-maintained school with a positive psychosocial climate creates an environment that helps learning achievements of pupils and increases self esteem among teachers and school staff. Providing clear rules about eating and drinking on the school premises.

7. Workplace health promotion for school staff
   Providing healthy food for school staff contributes to a healthy working environment. Including workplace health promotion.

8. Family and community involvement
   Nutrition programmes need to extend to the parents and families in order to have more impact. Also the community needs to be involved, for example by developing rules for shops that sell snacks and sweets within the vicinity of the school, or by designing a nutrition project that includes the parents and the community.

The most effective approach for school nutrition is including each of the eight components in a comprehensive programme. This can be elaborated into a school plan that fits the particular needs and demands from a school. The final aim of this strategy is to implement healthy nutrition in the overall school policy.

What does this approach mean for the professional?

A lot of patience, good timing and communication skills are required to make these plans work. One of the main challenges is a fundamental change in the perspective of the health promotion professional. Traditionally the health promotion worker and nutrition specialist have defined the nutrition problem, not the school itself. The expert explains, based on epidemiological data, that things are going wrong with healthy food habits of pupils. So we make an appeal to the interest of the school and ask them to take action. Now you can ask yourself: who is the owner of the problem?

Instead of the classical top-down approach where the expert decides what is important for a school, schools themselves are now invited to set their priorities. The best thing a professional can do is to support the school in clarifying their needs and to help them to get the best support they need. For the individual school doctor or school nurse, for local and national health promotion workers, this will be the major challenge for the coming years. We will need to focus more on processes than on contents, which requires a change in professional attitude.

The first and easiest step is by getting in direct contact with the most important setting for reaching young people: the school. There is increasing proof that this strategy will prove to have the most benefit in the end. That it will make learning and working in health promoting schools more fun. There are no problems, just possibilities.

Conclusion and recommendations

At the beginning of the new century the development of health promoting schools is at a crucial stage. This is true for the Netherlands and for Europe. We are only beginning to realise that a health promoting school actually benefits school improvement.

For health promotion professionals and nutrition specialists the development of a comprehensive school food policy with a central position for the individual needs of schools is capital. On the European level this development can be supported by meetings like these, and by developing joint projects where the effectiveness of these comprehensive school food programmes can be demonstrated, both in terms of improving the health status of children and in terms of school improvement. The big political issue concerning the health of young people in most or all of our countries is the prevention of overweight. Politicians have placed this high on their agendas. For us this offers the opportunity to develop our plans for a better school food policy. Prevention of overweight requires new thinking, including nutrition and physical activity as two important lifestyle issues. There is a great urgency to act, so let us offer our programmes and shared thinking in this process.

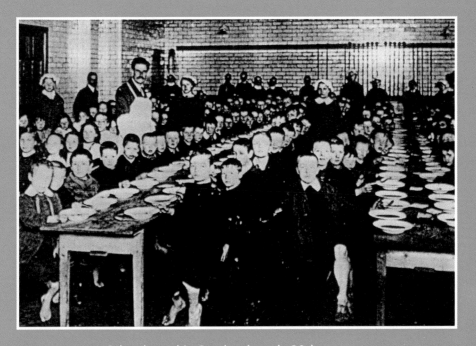

School meal in Scotland, early 20th century

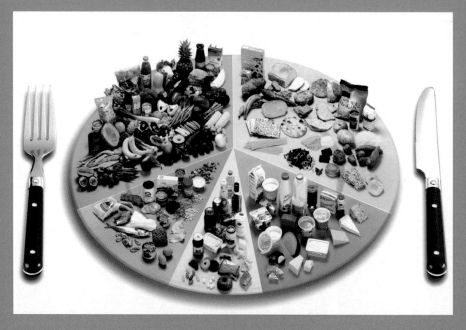

Balance of Good Health, concept from the Food Standards Agency,
visual from the British Nutrition Foundation, United Kingdom

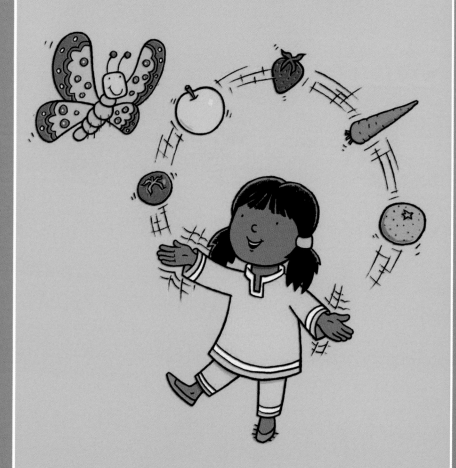

Eat five – fly high!

How many portions of fruit and vegetables do you eat a day?

Healthy Schools
© Crown copyright 2004
40260 1p 20k July 04 (COI)

School
Fruit and Vegetable
Scheme

Eat five - fly high, 5 a day, Department of Health, United Kingdom

Hungry for
Success:

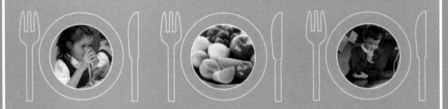

A Whole School Approach to School Meals in Scotland

Hungry for success, Scottish Executive Health Department,
United Kingdom

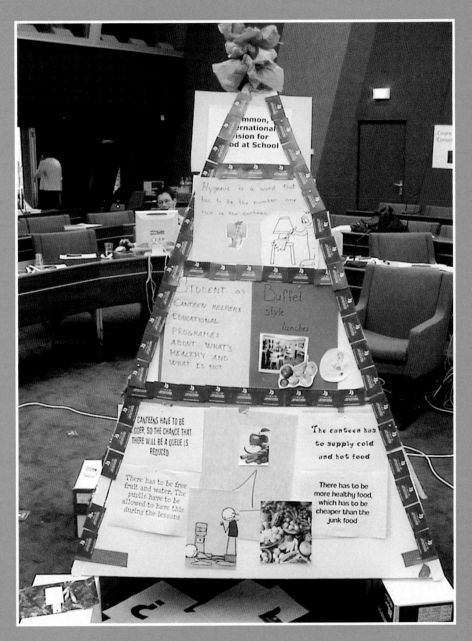

Young Minds pyramid, photo: Leif Glud Holm

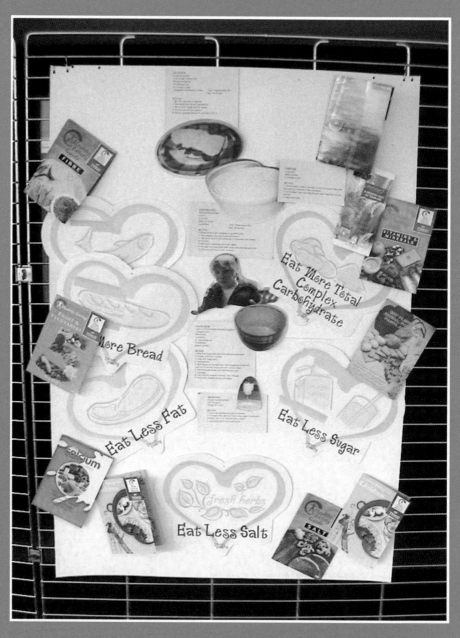

Young Minds poster, photo : Leif Glud Holm

Interactive CD-ROM: Discover Healthy Eating

B. Franchini, P. Graça, L. Sá, P. Queiroz, T. Silva, L. Rodrigues, MD. Vaz de Almeida

Faculty of Nutrition and Food Sciences - Portugal

Introduction

Discover Healthy Eating is an interactive CD-ROM for portuguese schoolchildren, aged 11-14 years old. This educational material was developed according to the school curriculum, by the *Faculty of Nutrition and Food Sciences* of Porto University in collaboration with the *Consumer Institute* and funded by the Programme Health XXI.

Objectives

The objectives of the CD-ROM are:

- to provide knowledge and a better understanding of food and nutrition sciences to schoolchildren;

- to stimulate an integrated and coordinated approach involving students, teachers and parents;

- to help schoolchildren to adopt healthy food habits and to be physically active.

Methodology

The design and graphics of the CD-ROM are centred around a fridge which displays several magnets on the door, each one corresponding to different sections. There are five sections: an interactive video, games, knowledge tests, a library and a competition (see fig. 1).

Video

The interactive video represents a day in the life of a young boy during which he goes to school, eats, practises physical activity and performs some households tasks. Throughout the day, the user can interact making different food choices for breakfast (see fig. 2) and other meals (see fig. 3) which will affect the boy´s ability to learn in the classroom and engagement in exercise (see fig. 4). A brief comment is made after each food choice. The user is also taught how to correctly store food items in the fridge (see fig. 5) and to understand how to use the food labels (see fig. 6).

Games

This section has three games where schoolchildren can develop their ability to learn and have fun at the same time. In the first game *Slice & Dice* (see fig. 7) the player has to construct a jigsaw puzzle. The second game is called *Gotcha* (see fig. 8) and the objective is for the player to score points by "catching" as many fruits, vegetables and soup as possible that fall from the top of the screen. However, the game ends if the player "catches" an alcoholic beverage. The third game *Match Up*, which has two levels, requires the player to find and match up two similar food items (see fig. 9).

Knowledge tests

The player knowledge on food and nutrition is tested (see fig. 10). The tests will not only evaluate their knowledge but will also help to improve it as the correct answers are given at the end of each test. Users can click on the library section to clear any doubts or queries they may have.

Library

The library is divided into various sub-sections that include for example information on nutrients, foodstuffs, food safety, tips on cooking and the importance of the meals. There is also a detailed glossary and links to related websites (see fig. 11).

Competition

The national competition entitled "The dish of my region" has two phases. The first, involves the pupil answering true or false questions on food and nutrition (see fig. 12), then, filling a form with personal details. The second, requires the pupil to be creative and prepare a recipe for a regional dish which can be presented in the form of a leaflet, poster or brochure.

Conclusion

This CD-ROM may constitute a very useful tool for teachers, parents and schoolchildren. It can also be incorporated into the school curriculum as well as being helpful for pupils to make healthy food choices outside the classroom.

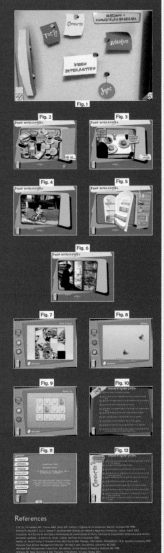

Fig. 1
Fig. 2 Fig. 3
Fig. 4 Fig. 5
Fig. 6
Fig. 7 Fig. 8
Fig. 9 Fig. 10
Fig. 11 Fig. 12

References

Interactive CD-ROM: Discover Healthy Eating, Porto University, Portugal

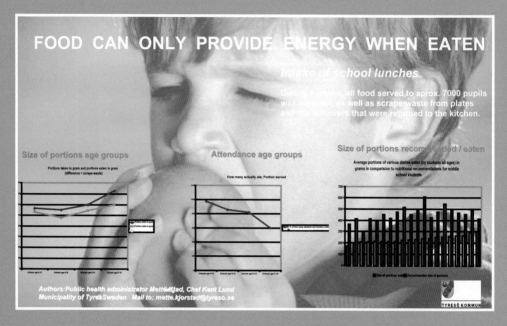

Food can only provide energy when eaten,
Municipality of Tyresö, Sweden

"DIME COMO COMES": A JOINT INITIATIVE BETWEEN THE CATERING SECTOR AND PUBLIC HEALTH NUTRITION

Aranceta J[1], PÈrez-Rodrigo C[1], Serra-Majem Ll[2], Delgado A[3]
[1] Community Nutrition Unit. Bilbao Department of Public Health (Spain); [2]Department of Preventive Medicine and Public Health. University of Las Palmas de Gran Canaria (Spain); [3] Department of Pediatrics. University of the Basque Country. Service of Pediatrics, Basurto Hospital, Bilbao (Spain).

INTRODUCTION: The objective of this paper is to analyse the contribution of school meals to food patterns of school-aged population and to evaluate the perceived quality of the service.

METHODS: 'Dime Como Comes' is a descriptive cross-sectional study carried out on a random population sample of children and young people (3-16 yr) having school meals in Spain. The study protocol included socio-economical data, food consumption and dietary habits at the school and out of the school. Information was collected by means of two questionnaires: one completed by children at school and a second one completed by the family at home

RESULTS: Valid response was collected from 322 children aged 3-16 years and 212 families, a response rate of 96,1% children and 63,3% of the families. 90% of children reported having a full meal for lunch. 70% of children having school meals perceived the portion served as adequate size. However 55% of boys and 40% of girls aged 12-16 years reported eating only half the serving. A dislike for the taste was the main reason (50%) followed by inadequate temperature (10%). In the school menus vegetables and fish were offered less frequently than other food groups. 45% of the sample had a midmorning snack and 81% an after-school snack. The overall food consumption pattern showed inadequate consumption of fruits and vegetables and a fair consumption for the dairy group.

DISCUSSION: This cross-sectional study provides interesting data on school meals in Spain. Catering companies supplying the service could contribute to increase the offer of fruit and vegetables in schools, inlcuding the availability of healthy foods as a choice for a mid-morning and/or after-school snacks particulary for children under 12 years.

* This survey had the logistic support of Sodexho Spain

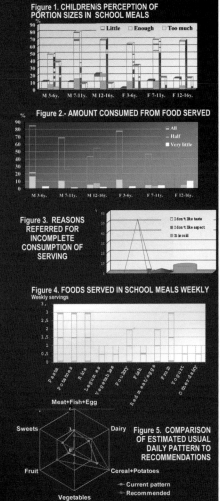

Figure 1. CHILDRENiS PERCEPTION OF PORTION SIZES IN SCHOOL MEALS

Figure 2.- AMOUNT CONSUMED FROM FOOD SERVED

Figure 3. REASONS REFERRED FOR INCOMPLETE CONSUMPTION OF SERVING

Figure 4. FOODS SERVED IN SCHOOL MEALS WEEKLY

Figure 5. COMPARISON OF ESTIMATED USUAL DAILY PATTERN TO RECOMMENDATIONS

PROJET LOCAL DE PRÉVENTION PRIMAIRE DE L'OBESITE DE L'ENFANT EN MILIEU SCOLAIRE DANS LE CADRE DU PROGRAMME NATIONAL NUTRITION SANTÉ (PNNS) FRANÇAIS :
Amélioration des habitudes alimentaires au Groupe scolaire de Ouistreham

CORES

Dr N. Lesplingard (directrice adjointe), J.M. Soulard (chargé de projet en éducation pour la santé),
Dr J.L.Veret (directeur), A. Pihan (éducatrice nutritionnelle), C. Chesnel (agent de développement en santé)
Dr D. Bouglé (médecin nutritionniste), S. Robert (diététicienne)

Comité Régional d'Education pour la Santé de Basse-Normandie
1 place de l'Europe – 14200 HEROUVILLE ST CLAIR
Tel:0231438361 Fax:0231438347 Courriel : cores.bn@noos.fr / cresbn14@hotmail.com

Ce projet de santé en milieu scolaire a pour objectif de permettre à l'enfant d'acquérir des habitudes alimentaires favorables à sa santé tout en développant sa liberté de choix et son autonomie. Il concerne 800 enfants âgés de 3 à 10 ans et associe l'ensemble des acteurs concernés par l'alimentation : les enfants eux-mêmes, les parents, les enseignants, les personnels de restauration et d'accompagnement de l'enfant, les élus. Il vise à créer des synergies pour élaborer entre acteurs locaux des solutions concrètes et innovantes aux difficultés rencontrés autour de l'alimentation.

Pour l'année scolaire 2002-2003, la démarche consistait à :
- Réaliser un état des lieux en donnant la parole aux enfants et adultes concernés par la qualité de vie à l'école : identifier des besoins, définir les ressources et les priorités d'action
- Elaborer des objectifs avec la communauté éducative selon les priorités locales
- Définir des critères d'évaluation

Pour l'année scolaire 2003-2004, la démarche consiste à :
- Mettre en place des interventions adaptées aux objectifs choisis
- Favoriser l'appropriation par les acteurs des changements de comportements et de la dynamique communautaire

2002-2003 : Nos objectifs de travail

✓ Promouvoir la consommation de fruits et légumes et diminuer la consommation d'aliments à forte densité calorique.
✓ Avoir des menus équilibrés et consommés réellement par les enfants au restaurant scolaire.

✓ Permettre la découverte de nouveaux mets et la familiarisation de l'enfant avec les fruits et les légumes

2003-2004 : Des interventions locales

Accompagner l'équipe de restauration scolaire pour :
✓ Augmenter de 15% la fréquence de légumes dans les menus mensuels.
✓ Permettre l'appropriation des orientations du Ministère de l'Education Nationale sur l'équilibre alimentaire.
✓ Augmenter la diffusion de fruits au moment du goûter du matin et aller vers une fréquence de 75% de goûters à base de fruits.
✓ Améliorer la présentation des légumes cuits et des crudités.

Discussion – Débat

L'année 2002-2003 a permis de mettre en application sur ce site les principes de la démarche communautaire pour une prévention de l'obésité des enfants à l'école : *accueil des préoccupations de chacun, élaboration d'une plate-forme de rencontre entre les acteurs, décloisonnement entre professionnels.*

L'état des lieux a mis en évidence une dévalorisation des fruits et des légumes dans l'horizon alimentaire des enfants. A partir de là, les enseignants, le CORES et les Agents Territoriaux Spécialisés des Ecoles Maternelles (ATSEM) ont élaboré des animations spécifiques visant la promotion des fruits.

En maternelle, les animations ont abouti *à généraliser une proposition de fruits au moment du goûter du matin. Ces fruits sont apportés par les parents.*

L'action communautaire a également permis *de résoudre des conflits entre acteurs.* Enfin, l'action permet de concentrer des énergies et des volontés jusqu'ici individuelles et qui de ce fait ne trouvaient pas toujours l'écho dans la collectivité.

Cette première année de recueil de données et d'élaboration du dispositif va aboutir à court terme à la mise en place d'actions portant sur le comportement de l'enfant, la relation adultes – enfants, et l'environnement de l'enfant.

Les actions porteront par la suite sur la promotion de l'activité physique, l'amélioration du sommeil. *Une évaluation d'impact sur 5 ans est en cours d'élaboration.* A partir des Indices de Masse Corporelle, il s'agit de faire un suivi comparatif et longitudinal de cohortes.

A plus long terme, ce travail vise à mettre en lien différents acteurs et à créer un réseau local de compétences et de volontés susceptibles de collaborer autour de diverses priorités de santé publique.

Projet local de prévention primaire de l'obésité de l'enfant en milieu scolaire dans le cadre du Programme National Nutrition Santé (PNNS) français, Comité Régional d'Education pour la Santé de Basse-Normandie, France

FINNISH SCHOOL MEALS OF 7TH-9TH GRADE PUPILS

Ulla-Marja Urho, M.Sc Dairy Nutrition Council, Helsinki, Finland, Pasilankatu 2, 00240 Helsinki, Finland.
Email: ulla-marja.urho@etl.fi

Background: In Finland since late 70's the school meals have been free to all pupils every school day from primary to high school level, ages 7-19.

There are guidelines for school meals, including advises about nutrition, composition of meals (main dish, bread with low-fat spread, vegetables, skimmed or low-fat milk and water) and environment of the canteen. Meals are served in school canteens by well trained personal, most of them community civil servants.

The importance of the school meal as a pedagogic tool to teach eating habits is emphasized as well the significance of increasing the consumption of vegetables, full corn bread and skimmed milk. No other drinks but milk and water should be served on a regular basis.

Objective: To describe the school meal patterns of Finnish pupils from the 7th to 9th grade, to analyse the differences in relation to recommendations on school lunches.

Methods: in the study of the year 2003 pupils (n=3028) from grades 7-9, in 12 different schools located around the country, answered a structured questionnaire right after the lunch break at class rooms. The study was now repeated for the fourth time.

Results year 2003

- 89% of pupils visited the school canteen
- 95% of pupils ate the main course (this is more than on previous studies)
- 50% of pupils drank milk and 47% ate the salad (these are less than on previous studies)
- 60% of pupils liked the main dish
- 60% of pupils used less than 10 minutes to eat the lunch

The model of school lunches

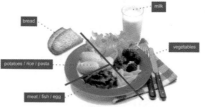

Conclusion: Skipping school meals appears not to be common among Finnish pupils, but only few of them eat a varied, balanced lunch. There are differences between boys and girls lunch models: boys eat more often the main course and drink the milk, girls eat more often the salad and bread. The pupils see the planned lunch as selection to make their own choices. Pupils drink more often milk when there are at least two types of milk (0% and 1,5% of fat) served.

Discussion: There are big differences between the realized school lunches in different schools. Making the guidelines mandatory and adding alternatives on salad, milk and bread could be means to improve the situation. Active follow-up and training of the canteen personal are important as well as the co-operation of all adults dealing with school lunches.

The combination of an average school lunch by the years of 1988, 1994, 1998 and 2003

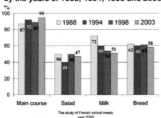

The study of Finnish school meals, year 2003

The average school lunch, year 2003

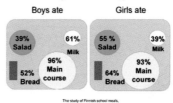

The study of Finnish school meals, year 2003

Finnish school meals of 7th - 9th grade pupils,
Dairy Nutrition Council, Finland

charlotte.lonfils@ulb.ac.be

L'UTILISATION DE L'INFORMATION DANS LE DÉVELOPPEMENT DE PROJETS EN ÉDUCATION NUTRITIONNELLE CHEZ LES JEUNES :
ENQUÊTE QUALITATIVE PRÉLIMINAIRE AUPRÈS D'ACTEURS DE TERRAIN.

C. Lonfils[1], T. Nguyen[2], D. Piette[1]

(1) Unité de Promotion Education Santé,
Ecole de Santé Publique,
Université Libre de Bruxelles
(2) Centre Local de Promotion de la Santé du Hainaut Occidental, Belgique

CONTEXTE Le point de départ de notre recherche est le constat d'une sous-utilisation de l'information lors du développement de projets par les intervenants de terrain.

OBJECTIF GÉNÉRAL Réaliser un état des lieux de l'utilisation de l'information auprès d'intervenants de terrain développant un projet en éducation nutritionnelle chez les jeunes.

OBJECTIFS SPÉCIFIQUES
- identifier les informations utilisées par les équipes de terrain
- mettre en évidence leurs besoins en matière d'informations
- étudier les éléments influençant l'utilisation de l'information
- identifier ce que les acteurs de terrain perçoivent comme informations utiles
- comprendre le travail de recueil d'informations effectué par les équipes de terrain.

MÉTHODOLOGIE Entretiens semi-directifs auprès de 12 intervenants de terrain actifs en éducation nutritionnelle, en Communauté française de Belgique.

RÉSULTATS La moitié des intervenants rencontrés a déclaré utiliser, de manière non régulière, des statistiques d'obésité chez les jeunes. L'utilisation de l'information intervient surtout lors de l'élaboration du projet. Parmi les différents éléments influençant l'utilisation de l'information fréquemment cités, les répondant évoquent : la visibilité des informations existantes ; le temps disponible ; le manque de formation, notamment pour interpréter les données statistiques ; le manque de données à caractère local ; la nécessité de fournir une interprétation claire des résultats ainsi que le travail en partenariat.

CONCLUSION Cette étude a permis d'identifier les informations utilisées par les répondants ainsi que différents éléments favorisant ou freinant cette utilisation. En outre, il apparaît que chez les intervenants rencontrés, les besoins ressentis en matière d'informations ne concernent pas des données spécifiques à une thématique mais plutôt un manque de données à caractère local. Des lacunes dans la formation des intervenants de terrain au niveau la définition de besoins en matière d'information et de l'interprétation des données ont également pu être mis en évidence.

Charlotte Lonfils
Ecole de Santé Publique – ULB
Route de Lennik 808, CP 596
1070 Bruxelles
Belgique
Tél.: 0032 (0)2 555 40 97

L'utilisation de l'information dans le développement de projets en éducation nutritionnelle chez les jeunes, Université Libre de Bruxelles, Belgium

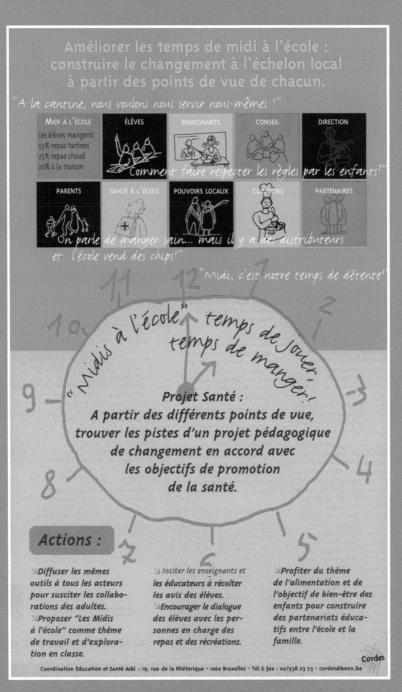

Améliorer les temps de midi à l'école, Coordination Education et Santé Asbl, Belgium

Developing healthy eating at school

Partnership between authorities and NGO's – the Danish experience

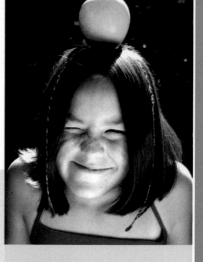

There is a growing awareness on the fact that partnerships between different stakeholders can be a powerful tool in promotion of healthy eating among citizens. Stakeholders can include authorities, practitioners, researchers, NGO's, private enterprises. The advantage is that through partnerships it is possible to obtain much greater effect of campaigns and policy implementations than stakeholders can obtain through individual efforts.

Partnerships have been investigated in many fields of policy making and public regulation including social policy, urban planning and international aid and development. Commercial partnerships have long been used to describe the cooperation between supplier and customer and these partnerships have already proven their effectiveness. The basic implication of a partnership is simply to do things together but the current understanding has been developed towards more committed partnerships.

This poster explores the Danish experience in a public NGO partnership project that aims at developing healthy school meal catering systems in Danish municipalities. In Denmark provision of school meals is not compulsory and hence it is for the municipalities and schools to decide whether school meal catering is to be provided. In most cases school meal catering does not exist and food is mostly provided by parents through an ordinary lunch box. However it is known that very often this lunch is not eaten. In stead a lot of sweets and soft drinks are consumed. Therefore the idea of a public provision of school meals enjoys support from parents and many politicians. The reason is that unhealthy eating habits can be influenced this way and busy parents have the possibility of avoiding preparing a lunch box. As a result many schools are open to the idea that school meals should be provided.

Ed. Mikkelsen, B.E., Skovby, K. & Christensen, L.M.

METHODS

The project was carried out in cooperation between the Danish research institute for Food Safety and Nutrition and the Danish Dietetic Association. The project aimed at carrying out an information campaign on healthy school meal catering targeted at the important stakeholders in and around the school environment.

OUTCOME

First an explorative research based on multiple qualitative case studies took place. Based on the findings a handbook was published and a series of workshops/meetings with practitioners were held. Key figures for dissemination of results

- 150 professionals participated in meetings across the country
- 250 copies of the handbook sold
- handbook published on the www.altomkost.dk site

The meetings have been very useful as a catalyst for creation of networks. Relations have been developed between kitchen staff, teachers, parents and school administrations.

REFERENCER

Balloch, S. & Taylor, M. Partnership working: policy and practice / edited by Sue Balloch and Marilyn Taylor, Bristol: Policy, 2001.

Christensen, L.M., Mikkelsen, B.E. & Jeppesen, Z (2002) Food for Children in Day-care Centers and Schools, Food Report 2002-9. Danish Veterinary and Food Administration & Danish Dietetic Association, Copenhagen.

Førde, B. (editor) Building partnerships: Lessons from Kenya and Zambia / Copenhagen 2000

Holker, H. & Flockhart, I. The case of Denmark: partnership project Aalborg: The European Research Unit, Aalborg University, 2001.- 471 s. - (European studies; 31) - (Series of occasional papers)

Håkansson, H. 1982: "Introduction - Technological innovation through interaction" (p 3-19), I Håkansson, H. (red.): Industrial Technological Development - A network Approach.

Håkansson, H. 1999: Product Development in Networks (p 475-498) in Ford, D. (ed) "Understanding Business Market"

Søndergård, B., Hansen, O.E. & Kerndrup, S. (1997): Cleaner production in a network perspective [Renere produktion i et innovationsperspektiv] i bogen Miljøreguleringen – tværfaglige studier] Holm, J., Kjærgård, B. & Pedersen, K. (editors), Roskilde University Publishing 1997

DISCUSSION

Strengths of partnerships

- More attention in the target group because of the joint efforts
- Easier access to the target group because a variety of communication channels are used
- Resources can be joined and as a result a minimum of critical mass necessary for carrying out ambitious projects can be obtained
- For NGO's the state involvement results in increased credibility
- For the authorities partnerships may lead to the effect that scarce resources can be used elsewhere
- Multidisciplinary approach resulting from the partners' different backgrounds can increase the quality of the outcome

Weaknesses of partnerships

- Partners risk to inherit "bad image" from the other partner
- NGO's are in some cases regarded as "narrow minded" and authorities may lose credibility as a result
- Are often very much dependant on individuals

Conditions for successful partnerships

- Open mindedness and active involvement from both parties is crucial for successful partnerships
- Accept of the partner's different motivation for participating in partnerships
- Accept of the fact that effective partnerships take time to build

The Danish Veterinary and food Administration
Danish Ministry of Food, Agriculture and Fisheries

 økonomaforeningen

Developing healthy eating at school, The Danish Veterinary and Food Administration, Denmark

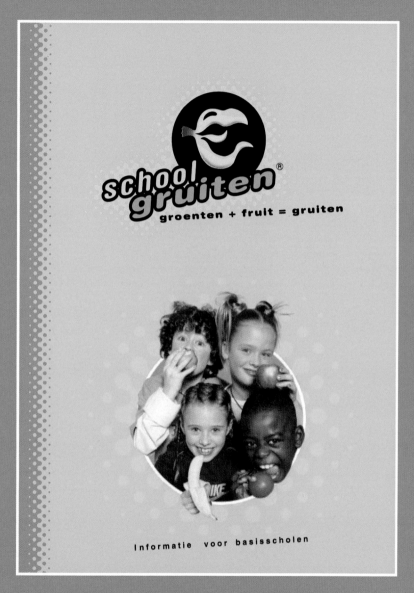

School gruiten, AGF Promotie Nederland, the Netherlands

Promoting good personal health care and healthy consumption habits through a good school climate

Jean-Claude VUILLE, Professor Emeritus of Social Paediatrics, Department of Public Health, Bern, Switzerland.

This paper describes the importance of the school climate or whole school effect and the evidence that it has the potential to influence health behaviours.

In view of a dramatic increase of the incidence of nutrition-related diseases, there is general agreement on the necessity of an active promotion of better nutrition habits. As is the case with many other lifestyle issues, the school is called upon to promote healthy nutrition, since the school is the only setting where the whole young population can be exposed to nutrition education programmes. However, the evidence of the effectiveness of nutrition education in school is scanty.

The paper presents data derived from a longitudinal evaluation of 'Health Teams at School', a general health promoting intervention in primary and secondary schools of the City of Bern. All but two of the public schools in the city participated in the project (n = 18), which extended over a period of five years (1997 to 2002). Process evaluation was mainly based on repeated interviews with principals and health co-ordinators (specially trained members of the teaching staff), whereas teacher and student (6th and 8th grade) questionnaires were used to collect data on outcome. The teacher questionnaires also contained questions on their health education practice.

As an outcome measure, the variable 'problematic eating behaviour' was derived from five questions in the student questionnaires:

- not eating breakfast regularly;
- not eating anything between breakfast and lunch;
- being aware of a problem with nutrition (eating too much, eating too little, behaviour suggesting bulimia, eating too much unhealthy and not enough healthy food);
- dieting;
- preferring not to eat anything if this were possible.

The evaluation of the effectiveness of health promotion activities was based on the observation that schools differed widely with respect to the following variables:

- experience of nutrition information in class reported by students;

- teacher reports on nutritional education given to their classes;
- providing healthy snacks and/or day-school with lunch;
- a standardised measure of the school climate derived from the student questionnaire.

Measuring the school climate

The pupil questionnaire on school climate had the following components:
- personal well-being at school (three questions);
- participation (three questions);
- relationships with teachers (eight questions);
- climate in class, peer relationship (six questions);
- bullying (three questions).

Climate score for each school was calculated on the basis of the answers of all pupils of the school.

Results

The following charts give examples of a range of variables and their relationship with 'problematic eating behaviour'

Prevalence of problematic eating behaviour (2002)

By age and gender

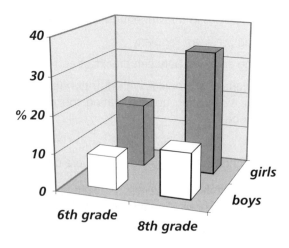

By ethnic background

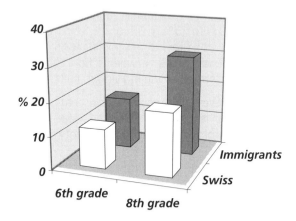

By social class

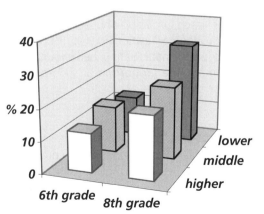

By school level (only secondary school)

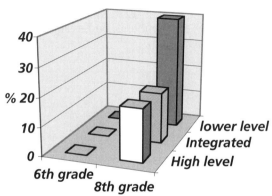

The proportion of problematic eating behaviour decreased between 1998 and 2002 from 20% to 15% in 6th grade, and from 29% to 25% in 8th grade. Available data do not provide any explanation for this unexpected phenomenon. Analyses of relationships between school factors and problematic eating behaviour were performed at the individual, the class, and the school levels.

1. Individual level: Children and adolescents, who felt comfortable at school, had significantly less eating problems. Reported experience of having received nutrition information in school was not consistently related to personal eating problems.

2. Class level: In those classes of 8th grade, where more than 70% of pupils reported to have had lessons on nutrition, the proportion of eating problems was lower than in other classes.

3. School level: None of the specific nutrition education activities of schools (day school with lunch, provision of healthy snacks, and a high proportion of teachers doing nutrition education) was statistically related to the proportion of students with problematic eating behaviour. However, in schools with a good general climate, the proportion of such problems was lower than in schools with a poor climate.

Conclusions

Statistically significant correlations are no proof of causal relationships, and non-significant correlations in a sample of n = 18 schools do not prove the absence of an effect. However, the observation that values of psychosocial determinants linked to eating behaviour were more positive in schools with a good climate suggests that efforts to create an unspecific healthy atmosphere may be more promising in the promotion of healthy food habits than specific nutrition interventions. Schools with a good climate also had lower consumption rates of tobacco, alcohol, and cannabis, and a higher proportion of students taking care of their own health.

Health and education intersectoral role of school nutrition and nutrition education

Cirila HLASTAN-RIBIC, Ministry of Health, Slovenia
Irena SIMCIC, Board of Education, Institute of Education, Slovenia

This paper reviews the policy and operational infrastructure for the provision of school food and demonstrates an intersectoral partnership model between education and health.

The Republic of Slovenia, although a country in transition, faces the same nutritional health problems as developed countries. The survey of the dietary habits of Slovenes (Koch 1997) shows that we overconsume foods with high content of fats (>44% E), that the share of carbohydrates is below the recommended levels (<40%), and that we under consume cereals, fruit and vegetables. The causes for this unsatisfactory situation in the field of nutrition are the same as elsewhere in Europe – changing lifestyles, diet and dietary habits, sedentary work, not enough physical activity – this all result in high incidence and prevalence of diet related chronic diseases in adult age.

Therefore healthy lifestyle and nutrition education have a start in early childhood in a family or in an environment where the child spends most of his /her daily time. And what is, beside a family, more appropriate than an educational environment?

Organised nutrition in educational institutions

There is a long tradition of organised nutrition in educational institutions in Slovenia. The reasons for organised school nutrition have changed over the years: in the 1970s and 1980s the aims of organised nutrition were directed towards improving the nutritional status of children and correction from nutritional deficiencies which originated in family nutrition. Today organised nutrition for children and youth represents an effective tool for the promotion and protection of health, improvement of bad dietary habits, nutritional education and also a help to the family where the number of family daily meals, due to our lifestyle, is decreasing rapidly. Slovenia is a country with a high rate of full time employed women – 46,2% of the employed population are women.

At the national level school nutrition in Slovenia is well supported by legal acts, policies, guidelines and recommendations in both education and health sectors. The framework Act on Education (1996) requires that every school must provide at least one school meal every day; there are important priorities in the National

Programme of Health Care of Slovenia (2000) in the field of health promotion and reducing the risk of nutrition related chronic diseases. These include the promotion of healthy diet, physical activity and nutrition education among young people.

Two formal bodies for the intersectoral collaboration of health and education have been set up in Slovenia: the Council for Food and Nutrition (a working group for preschool and school nutrition) within the Ministry of Health and the Programme Committee for Health within the Ministry of Education. Both bodies carry out, among other things, programme activities relating to the organisation of school nutrition and nutrition education curricula for primary schools. Both activities represent a vital part of the new Slovene Food and Nutrition Action Plan (in the final phase of preparation), co-ordinated by the Ministry of Health.

In the health sector many guidelines for the nutritional quality of school meals, safety and hygienic standards already exist and some of them are under review for the adaptation to new findings and other requirements.

In Slovenia, school building standards require that every school has kitchen facilities such as:

- own kitchen, preparing meals only for its own needs;
- central kitchen preparing meals for its own needs and other premises (other schools, kindergartens, secondary schools);
- distributing/satellite kitchen, distributing prepared meals from central kitchen.

The organisation of one school meal – morning meal/snack at the national level is part of the so-called National Programme, for which partial subsidising is provided by the Ministry of Education. Schoolchildren just pay for the price of foodstuffs composing the meal. Other meals such as lunch or breakfast are placed into the so-called economic, but non-profit programme. The whole price for the meal is paid by the schoolchildren. In primary schools approximately 97% of schoolchildren receive a morning meal/snack, 48% lunch and 7% breakfast. In kindergartens every child receives three daily meals (breakfast, lunch, afternoon snack). Only 20% of secondary schools prepare and offer one meal to the pupils.

The organisation of school nutrition requires qualified and experienced staff. A qualified cook is required if the school prepares at least 400 meals a day, and a catering manager is required if the school prepares 4,200 meals a day.

If the number of meals/snacks is bigger or smaller there is a justified suitable part for a certain working place. The catering manager organises all the meals in school. He or she must be an expert with the qualification of being a teacher of home economics or food technology engineer. The basic tasks of the catering manager are:

- planning the meals which satisfy the nutritional needs of pupils;
- organisation and surveillance of the working process in the school kitchen;
- taking care of cultural behaviour during the meals (appropriate dining rooms, hygienic system etc.);
- having contacts with parents, teachers and medical staff in cases of special nutritional needs (prescribed medical diets for children – diabetes, coeliac disease, food allergies);
- training of kitchen staff in the field of nutrition, food safety and hygiene.

In most schools a person who is the catering manager also teaches the subject home economics. The subject home economics is a regular/obligatory subject in Slovene primary schools and is taught from 5th to 9th class. Nutrition themes and education take the main part of teaching hours within this subject. In lower classes (one to four) nutrition is a cross-curricular subject.

Future activities

As Slovenia is a country which already has a very good organisation and access to school nutrition, the main priority is now to preserve this standard. In the draft of the Food and Nutrition Action Plan of Slovenia, co-ordinated by the Ministry of Health, some priorities in the field of nutrition in schools are:

- the updating of present nutrition guidelines for prepared meals;
- preparation of new food based dietary standards for school meals;
- nutrition surveillance;
- review of nutrition curricula;
- permanent education and training of all teaching staff for healthy eating and physical activity.

The same priorities shall be addressed to secondary/middle schools – the goal is to assure the same standard of organised nutrition to our school population aged 15 to 18 years as that which exists in primary schools.

Discussion: Whole school approach

The facilitator Maria Vaz de Almeida gave delegates the opportunity to raise issues on the theme of the whole school approach.

On the subject of sharing good practice ......

Aileen Robertson (WHO). Based on the presentation of Goof Buijs, it seems to me that case studies are useful and there is probably a need to submit case studies to WHO for sharing on our website.

Aileen Robertson (WHO). Another issue that concerns me is advertising and marketing: are schools educating young people about this?

Ian Young (rapporteur) referred to the training manual being produced in Scotland entitled 'Growing through Adolescence' (Poster 7) which explores the psycho-social issues, including media influences, in relation to healthy eating. He explained that it would be made available in 2004 to other countries that wished to consider adapting it for their own use and that discussions were ongoing with WHO about this.

On the subject of school climate.......

Danish Delegate. A question for Jean-Claude Vuille. What is a good school climate?

Jean-Claude Vuille. (Switzerland). An operational response would be: do people feel well? Are there low levels of bullying in the school? Are there good relationships between pupils and teachers in the school? As to how you create a good school climate: if the health promoting school activities are integrated into general school development it seems to be important. Also schools need to set their own agenda and priorities.

On the subject of the curriculum........

Stefka Petrova (Bulgaria). Which approach is most effective to integrate nutrition education best? Is it through different subjects or in a special subject?

Irina Simcic (Slovenia) explained that in her country they had developed a subject of healthy lifestyles.

Mette Kjörstad (Sweden) pointed out that the school's core task is education and therefore linking health issues to this is the key.

Cristine Deliens (Belgium) referred to a project 'Art d'écoles' integrating a creative arts approach to food and health in the classroom.

Mark Karaczun (England) referred to a project developed by 'Sustain' in England on developing a food policy, which drew on many subjects in the curriculum such as media studies, art and history.

Jenny Woolfe (England) referred to the project 'Getting to grips with grub'. This offers practical support to young people so that they have the knowledge and skills to cope when they eventually live independently (see interview for more information).

On wider policy issues.......

Ursula O'Dwyer (Ireland) explained that Ireland was considering the issue of advertising control in relation to targeting young people with potentially unhealthy products. She explained that in relation to meal provision in schools there was no statutory provision except for the children of low income families. She stated that where free meals are available teachers often report better behaviour in pupils.

Bauke Houtsma (The Netherlands). As a school principal he took the view that it was important to link school quality generally with the health promoting school and the promotion of healthy eating. These were not separate processes.

We decide what we eat: active involvement of students in developing school meal policies

Bjarne Bruun Jensen, Professor, Danish University of Education, Copenhagen.

Bjarne Jensen explores concepts such as participation, knowledge and nutrition in this challenging presentation. He explains the need to place healthy eating in a context which takes account of the wider socio-cultural and environmental realities of our lives.

Introduction

The title of my presentation deals with the involvement of young people in educational processes and therefore I will begin with discussing two pressing general questions in the area of health education. Both are relevant in relation to the overall aim of health education and promotion and therefore also for schools' work with nutrition: the development of pupils' abilities to influence their own life and their ability to influence their living conditions – their 'action competence'.

The first question to be discussed concerns the widespread notion that target groups should be directly involved in the processes of health education. This trend may be clearly seen in relation to teaching in schools. The second question concerns what kinds of knowledge or insights about healthy schools pupils should acquire during health education. Is it perhaps the case that knowledge in the field of health education and promotion is not really that important, and that the central matter is to strengthen the self-confidence and commitment of the pupils and to contribute to the clarification of their values, and such like?

This paper argues that the role and content of knowledge must be subjected to critical analysis, and must be related closely to the aims of health education. Moreover, if these aims are not formulated carefully enough, then an attempt must be made to do this if the discussion about knowledge is to be moved forwards. In connection with the discussion of both these questions, models and systematic approaches will be explored that can help to structure the discussion of the educational aspects of these themes.

I wish to make the case that we need to distinguish between different forms of participation in health education and promotion. Furthermore, participation might focus on a number of different questions in health education and therefore it makes no sense to describe a project as participatory or the opposite.

There are many reasons that we may give to justify the involvement of the pupils in their own learning. These include ideas such as ownership, intellectual freedom, democracy and equity. In addition there is an ethical case based on the need to involve participants in processes that are centrally related to their own lives. Most contemporary projects within health education aim explicitly, in some way or another, in involving the 'target group' as active agents. This current trend is the surface manifestation of a number of different theoretical justifications, and at the same time, poses a variety of new challenges to teaching in these topics.

This desire to involve the participants is evident both in educational theory and educational practice. For example, all the school co-ordinators at an evaluation seminar within the Danish Network of Health Promoting Schools agreed to the statement that if one does not succeed in involving pupils from the start, one might as well forget all about developing their action competence and empowerment (Jensen 1998). In this case, the motivation was mostly related to effectiveness, and influenced to a large extent by experiences indicating that pupils' participation is the most decisive precondition for arousing and developing their involvement, and for the knowledge gained by the pupils to be applicable at all. Thus, on the basis of this experience, action competence and empowerment are abilities to be actively acquired, and not just skills to be simply 'passed on' by someone, and passively received.

However, this project – and the concluding evaluation seminar – also revealed that there is a tendency to conceive of, and refer to, pupils' influence and pupil involvement on a very vague and general level, and that these terms often have diverse and ambiguous meanings. Phrases such as 'starting with the pupils', 'linked to the pupils', 'co-determination', 'influence, 'user involvement', 'co-influence', 'co-responsibility', 'participation' and 'involvement' are often used more or less haphazardly, without careful definition, in discussions.

For these reasons the example of 'The Health Promoting School' project points to the need to qualify the concept of participation itself as a precondition for further discussion and development. These tendencies are not only found within schools, but also in the broader debate about education in our society.

Involvement – different forms!

First we can talk about different forms of participation. Pupils' participation is often equated with 'pupil determination', that is, the idea that the 'target group' should formulate its visions more or less unaided, work out a plan of action and set about 'changing the world'. In this connection it has to be said that as far as schools are concerned not many of these projects succeed. Instead, many experiences with the involvement of pupils indicate that it is really necessary for the teacher to be involved in the process and the dialogue as a responsible, though respectful, partner. When trying to develop their visions and attitudes, pupils need a 'sparring partner' who can challenge them and with whom they can try out their views.

As a development from a model of the environmental psychologist Roger A. Hart, who is well known for his books on 'Children's Participation' (Hart, 1992, 1997), I wish to propose a matrix model of participation.

Figure 1. Participation matrix. Operationalising the concept of participation

	In the project	Selecting the theme	Investigation	Vision/ Goals	Actions	Evaluation/ Follow up
Pupils' suggestions Common decisions						
Pupils' suggestions Pupils' decisions						
Teachers' suggestion Common decisions						
Teachers inform Pupils accept						
Teachers' decisions told clearly to pupils						

The bottom level of the figure (non-participation) has been included to make it quite clear that in some cases, for one reason or another, participation is not possible.

There follow four levels of co-determination, which, although the boundaries between them may be fluid, represent different ideal types. The first refers to a situation in which the teacher puts forward a proposal that is accepted by the students without much discussion. One may of course quite reasonably ask whether this has anything to do with involvement. The next three levels are distinguished from each other by a combination of (1) who puts up an idea or proposal for discussion, and (2) who actually takes the final decision.

These three levels have been important in the school context, as there is sometimes the implicit presumption that any principle of involving pupils excludes almost per se the teacher presenting a proposal as the basis for discussion.

The important point to focus on here is the subsequent dialogue and discussion, which must be carried out with the 'target group' (determining the content and premises of a 'respectful' dialogues of this kind would call for another article, and will not be treated further at this point).

The top level of the matrix is inspired by Hart, who places 'Child-initiated, shared decisions with adults' at the top of his ladder model, even higher than 'Child-initiated and directed'. In the school context, this priority stresses how necessary it is for the teacher to appear as a responsible adult with his/her own opinions when involved in projects built around pupil participation. The more the pupils themselves are involved, the more important, presumably, it will be for the teacher to be visible and to play an active role in the discussions. Hart concludes his essay in the following way (Hart, 1992, p. 44):

"Productive collaboration between young and old should be the core of any democratic society wishing to improve itself, while providing continuity between the past, present, and the future".

When using this model in connection with health education, different weightings may be given to the three highest levels in terms of priority and quality, and this will, moreover, probably vary from project to project as well as from teacher to teacher. The aim of Figure 1, therefore, is to systematise the discussion of participation in relation to a particular health education project rather than to indicate a ranking order as such. Consequently, the three upper levels should be described as different forms rather than different levels of participation.

Furthermore, an actual project will involve a particular way of reacting to the questions that appear along the horizontal axis. The number and type of themes presented will naturally vary from project to project, and it is therefore important to note that, in any given project, there will be different types of participation in relation to different areas of decision. In other words, the aim is not to establish an ideal model for health education activities, according to which involvement is to be interpreted and applied in specific ways. On the contrary, it is important to insist that the partners who are working together (which also includes the 'target group') should spend some time discussing how and in relation to which questions and decisions they will include the involvement aspect. Figure 1 might be able to help in this respect.

The matrix reflects the assumption that participation, as well as its educational value, is context bound. And the context might consist of a number of factors:

- the character of the project;
- the personality of the teacher;
- the 'preparedness' among the students;
- which stakeholders are involved.

In conclusion, the crucial element is not who originally gets the idea to do something but rather the dialogue which follows and makes it possible for different stakeholders to take ownership.

Four dimensions of action-oriented knowledge

According to the resolution from the first international Health Promoting Schools Conference, the overall aim of the work of the school is that pupils develop skills and competencies that enable them to act in relation to their own lives and the conditions in their environment. In this connection, the resolution states that the overall aim is the development of the pupils' 'Empowerment and action competence', and it is further stated that "…The Health Promoting School improves young people's abilities to take action and generate change". In other words, action and change are the central concepts here.

Working with students as active participants in health education and promotion does not make health 'content' superfluous. Instead, it has to be re-thought from an action perspective. This point of departure has great consequences for the kind of knowledge that will be the focus of planning, implementing and evaluating the teaching and learning.

Four different aspects of action-oriented knowledge can be illustrated using the model in Figure 2. The four dimensions illustrate different perspectives on the types of knowledge through which a given health topic such as nutrition can be viewed and analysed.

Figure 2. Four dimensions of action-oriented knowledge

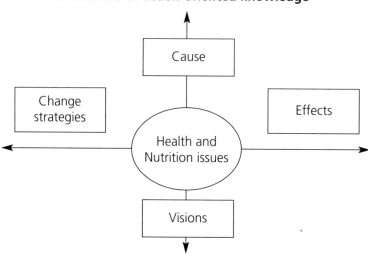

1st dimension: What kind of problem is it? - Knowledge about effects

The first dimension deals with knowledge about the existence and spread of health problems. This type of knowledge can, for example, be about the consequences of a given behaviour (such as too much fat in our diet). This knowledge is important, as it is the kind that awakens our concern and attention, and creates the starting point for a willingness to act. So this type of knowledge can be one of the prerequisites for developing action competence. However, this form of knowledge is mainly of a scientific nature and, on its own, risks contributing to developing concern and action paralysis among students as it gives no explanation for these problems, let alone how we can contribute to solving them.

2nd dimension: Why do we have the problems we have? - Knowledge about root causes

The next aspect deals with the 'cause' dimension of our health problems. Such causes include the associated social, cultural and economic factors behind our behaviour, and might include questions such as the effect of advertisements on our eating behaviour, the price of healthy food versus 'junk food', and the availability of healthy food in the school canteen etc. This knowledge belongs mainly in the sociological, cultural and economic areas. Explanations about the increasing inequalities in health are to be found within this area.

3rd dimension: How do we change things? - Knowledge about change strategies

This dimension deals with both knowledge about how to control one's own life and how to contribute to changing living conditions in society. How do we change surrounding structures, for example in a school, in a community or in our family? Who do we turn to, and who could we ally ourselves with? This type of knowledge also includes knowing how to encourage co-operation, how to analyse power relations, and so on. It is often to be found within psychological, political and sociological studies, and is central to an action-oriented health education and promotion activity. How do students go about it if they want to establish a canteen at the school and how are young people able to influence the 'eating pattern' in the family (e.g. if they want more time together with their parents when they have dinner, etc.).

4th dimension: Where do we want to go? - Knowledge about alternatives and visions

The fourth dimension deals with the necessity of developing one's own visions. Seeing real possibilities for forming and developing one's dreams and ideas for the future in relation to one's own life, work, family and society, and having the support and surplus energy to realise them, is an important pre-requisite to the motivation and ability to act and change.

The four dimensions in Figure 2 show that traditional health information would be placed along the first dimension axis: the one which is concerned with knowledge of effects of health conditions. The scientific approach is dominant in this type of information and the focus is on students attaining knowledge about the serious health problems that might affect them, how quickly such problems are evolving, which behaviour leads to risks of illness, etc.

This type of knowledge is not necessarily action promoting, especially when it stands alone. Indeed such knowledge can create a great sense of worry and, if this type of knowledge is not followed up by knowledge about causes and strategies for change, then it can be associated with breaking down commitment and contributing to action paralysis. We need to insist on including causal analyses and ways of producing change within health education.

Therefore knowledge based aspects should be thoroughly considered in the light of an action and change perspective. Participatory and action-oriented health education and nutrition education is not without basic knowledge and insight: on the contrary, it demands that a new 'landscape' of extensive and coherent knowledge and insight is being developed. This creates important demands and challenges for future teachers, who should be both in a position to fulfil the consultant role and, furthermore, from his/her own experience and talent be able to perceive today's health conditions from an inter-subject and action-oriented point of view.

The notion of 'nutrition' in a health promoting school

Finally, a few comments will be made about the issue of nutrition in health education. Many schools from the Danish network of health promoting schools have emphasised the broad WHO definition of health in their projects. This definition implies that health is about more than the absence of disease; it is also about life quality and mental an social well-being. From projects dealing with nutrition and food, the model in figure 3 has been developed:

Figure 3.

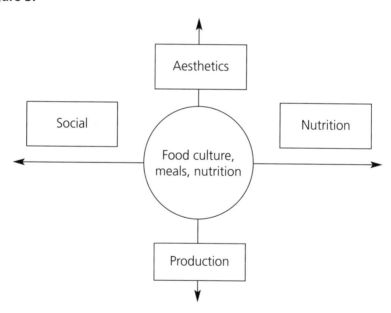

The figure illustrates the concept, with which students and teachers have worked in the area of eating habits/food/nutrition. The area is much broader that the traditional and scientific-oriented 'nutrition' concept. Nutrition is viewed only as one dimension of food quality. Another dimension deals with aesthetics (how does the food taste, how does it smell, how does it look etc.). This dimension is considered as very important by students and teachers while working with an approach, which is based on and inspired by the WHO definition of health. The third dimension is about the social environment. How do we 'organise' our meals – at home, in schools, with friends etc.? And finally, a fourth dimension deals with the conditions under which our food is produced. It includes considerations about animal welfare in the industrial farming industry, pollution of the environment, the quality of the worksite environment for the employers etc.

This broader approach – as well as the model itself - has been developed by teachers and students who have been participating actively in 'nutrition' projects at health promoting schools. At the same time the model is currently also used by teachers as a framework for involving students in discussion and debates about good food quality.

This approach is also mirrored in the 'Young Minds' project where young people are using IT to collaborate on health issues across cultural borders (www.young-minds.net). In the 'Young Minds' project leading up to a big health promoting school conference in 2002, students from four countries collaborated on the issue of nutrition. Within this collaboration it was obvious that the young people viewed health and nutrition in the light of the more positive WHO definition. For instance, one of the classes developed an 'alternative nutrition pyramid' where the two most important 'layers' in the pyramid were 'Better quality of food' and 'Cheerful friendly atmosphere during meals'.

From these experiences it is clear the words and concepts we use are crucial for the way health is viewed in school practice. It is also obvious that the words we often use in health education and health promotion have been developed by the natural sciences and consequently they might militate against the more open and broad notions that are central to a health promoting school approach. Instead of nutrition projects it is perhaps more recommendable to deal with projects about 'food, culture and the environment' – if we want to collaborate with young people and to involve them in the dialogue as genuine participants.

References

Currie, C., Hurrelmann, K., Settertobulte, W., Smith, R., & Todd, J. (2000). *Health and Health Behaviour among Young People. International Report* (Copenhagen, WHO Regional Office for Europe).

Danish Ministry of Education (1995a). *Curriculum Guide for Health and Sexual Education and Family Knowledge* (Ministry of Education, Copenhagen).

Danish Ministry of Education (1995b). *Ministry of Education Consolidation Act No. 55 f 17 January 1995.*

Due, P., Holstein, b. & SAWITZ, A. (1998) *Health Behaviour in School-aged Children: Population, Methods and Answer-distributions, Denmark* (University of Copenhagen, Institute of Public Health).

Hart, R.A. (1992). *Children's Participation: From Tokenism to Citizenship* (UNICEF International Child Development Centre. Spedale degli Innocenti. Firenze, Italy).

Hart, R.A. (1997). *Children's Participation. The Theory of Involving Young Citizens in Community Development and Environmental* Care (London: Earthscan Publications).

Hillcoat, J., Forge, K., Fien, J. & Baker, E. (1995). "I think it is really great that someone is listening to us …". *Environmental Education Research*, Vol. 1, pp. 159-171.

Hillgaard, P. & Jensen, B. B. (2000). We decide – a case story from Gandrup School. In Jensen, B.B. (ed.). *Action, Learning and Change. Case Stories from the Danish Network of Health Promoting Schools* (Komiteen for sundhedsoplysning, Copenhagen) pp. 24-48.

Jensen, B.B. (1997). A case of two paradigms within health education. *Health Education Research*, Vol 2, No. 4, pp. 419-28.

Jensen, B.B. (2000). Health knowledge and health education in relation to a democratic health promoting school. *Health Education,* Vol. 100, No 4, pp 146-153.

Jensen, B. B. & Schnack, K. (1997). The action competence approach in environmental education. *Environmental Education Research*, Vol. 3, No. 2, pp. 163-178.

Jensen, B. B. & Simovska V. (2003). *Young-minds.net/lessons learnt.* Danish University of Education.

Settertobulte, W., Jensen, B.B. & Hurrelmann, K. (2001). Alcohol consumption among young Europeans. World Health Organization, Regional Office for Europe, Copenhagen, 2001.

Simovska, V. & Kostarova-Unkovska, L. (1998). Conceptual framework for the Macedonian Network of Health Promoting Schools. In: SIMOVSKA, V. (ed.). *The European Network of Health Promoting Schools in Macedonia* (Faculty of Philosophy, Institute of Psychology, Skopje, Macedonia).

WHO (1986). *The Ottawa Charter for Health Promotion* (WHO Regional Office for Europe, Copenhagen).

WHO (1987). Regional Office for Europe, Technical Secretariat of the ENHPS (1997). Conference resolution. "*The Health Promoting School - an investment in education*, health and democracy". First Conference of the European Network of Health Promoting Schools. International Planning Committee of the European Network of Health Promoting Schools: WHO Regional Office for Europe/European Commission/Council of Europe. Copenhagen.

YOUNG MINDS (2002). www.young-minds.net (the website was visited 30 September 2003).

Eating at school: The school and parents as partners – Utopia or reality?

Patricia MELOTTE and Christophe CONTENT, Parents' Association "Clair-Vivre" Pre-Primary and Primary School, Belgium

This paper offers a real life insight into some of the issues, which have to be addressed when parents take the initiative in bringing about change in a school.

Introduction

A group of parents, interested in the issue of eating behaviour at school, organised a large-scale survey of parents and teachers. The vast majority of teaching staff and parents perceived this as a positive initiative. Presentation of the results made it possible to forge contacts with some of the school's teachers who had already attempted to introduce some innovative ideas in this field. Links were also established with parents having professional experience in the spheres of dietetics and catering for large administrative organisations, which will be extremely useful when following up the lines of action emerging from the survey.

The Clair-Vivre school

Clair-Vivre is an elementary school, which opened in 1964 at Evere in the Brussels-Capital region. Since its foundation it has constantly claimed as its own and applied the principles developed by the French pedagogue Célestin Freinet. Today the school has some 900 pupils from 1st grade nursery to 6th grade primary, on three separate sites: 'Clair-Vivre Centre', 'Geminal' and the 'Complexe'.

At Clair-Vivre, learning is based on children's own experience. The school's educational approach is aimed at developing happy, fulfilled, independent individuals, capable of expressing themselves, communicating, working together, showing creativity and assuming their responsibilities as members of society. In view of this pedagogic approach, the parents' association considered itself entitled to look to the school to develop responsible consumer attitudes, in particular regarding eating habits, in its pupils.

Teachers and pupils work together in the school. The adults encourage the children to take a significant share of responsibility and to agree among themselves the rules governing their community life. The children have three opportunities to make their voices heard:

- the Class Council, which meets once a week and brings together all pupils in the same class;
- the School Council, on which each class has a democratically elected representative;
- the Enlarged School Council, including representatives of all partners within the school.

As a result of Clair-Vivre's pedagogic approach, the parents are more involved, albeit indirectly, in their children's learning processes. It was this door deliberately left open by the school and necessary to its pedagogic processes that gave the Environment Group the impression that it would be welcome as a purveyor of projects and objectives in line with the school's teaching philosophy.

The parents also exert an influence through two other bodies: firstly, through the participatory board, which brings together representatives of the education authority, teaching staff, parents and local social, cultural and business circles, and through the parents' association, which includes various activity groups. As is frequently the case, only a minority of parents takes a truly active role in school life. The vast majority lack the time or the desire to become involved, or quite simply chose to send their children to this school because it was local.

Emergence of the project

When the Environment Group first raised the issue of healthy eating at a meeting of the enlarged school council in 2002, it based its arguments on a number of observations:

- some teachers encouraged children to bring sweets or snacks to school to celebrate a festive occasion or used these as a means of reward;
- the school sold lemonade as a lunchtime drink, without this being clearly mentioned in the food and drink accounting records;
- many parents were dissatisfied with the quality and composition of hot school meals.

Having voiced its surprise at the indirect encouragement of behaviour incompatible with a responsible, healthy approach to food choices and its desire to propose solutions for improving school meals, the parents' association then asked a fundamental question: did the school consider itself concerned and deem the subject worthy of its attention?

The reply was negative: the school's representatives thought it a matter not for the school but for the parents. The Environment Group's concerns were more-over deemed to be of marginal importance, and the school's attitude was systematically to play down the issue as a mere question of 'going organic'. Confronted with what resembled a 'dialogue of the deaf', the group decided to legitimate its concerns and give them a factual basis by drawing up an exhaustive questionnaire to be sent to all parents and the entire teaching staff. Their aim was to persuade others of the importance of their objectives, but also to achieve representativeness, conveying the wishes of a majority of the parents. They assumed that other parents were probably asking themselves the same questions. This made it appropriate to conduct a detailed survey covering the many aspects of the issue, since the group could not disregard differing opinions or levels of satisfaction in such matters nor fail to take account of criteria such as the amount individual parents were prepared to spend on their child's school meals.

Whom to target with the questionnaire?

The group's spontaneous initial response was to target the parents, not the children, although they are the direct consumers and hence in a better position to give an opinion on school meals. This decision was partly due to the fact that the initiative originated with the parents' association, which made it logical to involve the parents. It was also influenced by the belief that parents play an important role in what their children eat and in shaping their eating habits, although children are also entitled to a say, especially as they grow older. Nor did the Environment Group want to tread on the teachers' toes, wishing to leave them entirely free to inculcate healthy eating precepts as they saw fit. Lastly, it was important to know whether the parents had particular expectations of the school.

We also considered it essential to consult the teaching staff, a category, which we extended to youth workers, to compare their opinions with the parents' reactions on the same issues and also to obtain an insight into the real situation on the ground, since most of the teachers supervised school meals. It must be admitted that, doubtless as a result of the initial very negative reactions, the group's decision was influenced more by a desire not to offend the teachers' susceptibilities, rather than the hope of establishing a partnership. If the teachers had not participated, the results of the survey would have been perceived as an attempt to impose the parents' way of thinking. The question of consulting the children was raised again at a later stage, but the group postponed taking a decision on this subject in view of the huge workload involved in analysing the responses to the survey.

Field of study

Although the group originally intended to limit the number of questions, since it wished to impose on the parents and teachers only once, the final questionnaire contained 24 questions some of which included subsidiary questions and multiple-entry tables. The questions were designed to sound out the following: degree of interest in the issue of healthy eating at school; opinions on the food and drink proposed by the school not only for lunch but also as snacks; the reasons underlying choices and behaviours; and hence the parents' beliefs and wishes as to the school's role: opinions on various proposals requiring a greater physical effort or a bigger financial investment from the school or the parents.

The teaching staff were also asked about how the school meals functioned; their current participation in the awareness-raising effort; their interest in such matters, any measures taken in practice - where? how? by whom? at what frequency? - their requirements as to teaching materials and, lastly, their opinion on the initiative.

Presentation of the results

We shall not go into details of the results of the survey here. It can nonetheless be noted that their analysis showed that 90% of parents and teaching staff were concerned about the variety, balance and quality of school meals. The parents often mentioned the importance of a friendly, calm atmosphere in the school canteen. At Clair-Vivre one child out of every four takes school meals. The price of a full, hot lunch is two euros. Three-quarters of the parents of children taking school meals said they were satisfied with the quality and variety. However, 80% of the teachers supervising school meals thought they lacked variety, appeal and balance. With regard to snacks, 99% of children brought something from home because their parents wanted to control what their children ate, did not trust the quality of snacks sold by the school or considered them too expensive. The parents acknowledged that they gave their children too many sweets and biscuits and that they should give more preference to fresh or dried fruit and dairy products. Nearly 90% of parents and teachers thought the school should play a role in teaching good eating habits. Two-thirds of teachers already applied awareness-raising measures in the classroom. Nearly 80% of both parents and teachers wanted the school to impose restrictions on bringing certain types of food and drink to school. However, 58% of parents wanted the school to ban certain foodstuffs, whereas only 10% of teachers subscribed to such bans.

At the meeting to present the results to the parents and teachers, the audience was allowed to interrupt the presentation with questions at any time, in order to foster an interactive exchange of views.

Annex 1: School and teachers

What parents suggest

Food concerns:

- a quiet environment while having lunch is a must;
- good nutritional balance: sugar, fats and proteins;
- try to adapt to the pupil's tastes and eating habits;
- traceability and origins of products.

Why does my child eat school dinners:

- main meal is at midday not in the evening;
- parent/s return home late and has/ve no time to cook.

Why does my child bring packed lunches to school:

- the child is faddy, has not enough appetite to eat a hot meal at lunchtime;
- bad quality of school dinners, lack of confidence in supplier of school dinners;
- extra-school activities during lunch breaks.

Annex 2: Snacks and drinks

What parents say

Why bring snacks (99%) instead of buying at school:

- more variety;
- avoid transfer of money in school bags;
- less packaging waste by using reusable washable containers;
- fits the child's food and drink tastes;
- healthier and better value for money than what the school offers.

Why bring drinks from home (85%) rather than buying at school:

- bad quality of drinks sold at school (fizzy drinks);

- less packaging waste (reusable bottles vs bottles thrown away);
- against fizzy drinks products.

Why buy drinks at schools (15%):
- lighter school bags;
- avoid drinks that open up and spill in school bags.

How can the figures be translated into action?

The question is now to move beyond the results, that is to say obtain their acceptance as such and use them as a basis for determining lines of action. How can the expectations of those who want immediate results and visible, tangible actions straight away be reconciled with the views of those who first want to bring about a change of attitudes, to work behind the scenes? Is the solution to strike a balance between the two? And if so, how? With which potential partners? External partners or internal partners such as the school nurse? Account must also be taken of the problems posed by issues of authority, responsibility and competition.

Some parents' occupations - dietician - or experience - maintaining the 'cold chain' in a hospital context - could prove very helpful during future negotiations with the school meals provider concerning amendments to the contractual conditions. A further example was one teacher's testimony about the failure of a previous experiment with bringing healthy snacks to school. The formation of small discussion groups on themes of special interest to certain individuals was another possible line of action proposed by the Environment Group. Seeking the children's own opinion was naturally another key component of the lines of action proposed, and the teachers agreed to take charge of the co-ordination aspects.

Conclusion

Parental involvement in the issue of healthy eating at school should be perceived as one example of how parents can participate in the school community's day-to-day life. The Environment Group also believes that healthy eating principles and habits are part of the vital lessons to be taught in school with a view to children's integration into society. Although the teachers welcomed the survey, it was organised entirely at the parents' initiative. The initial links forged between parents and teachers at the meeting to present the results constitute the beginnings of a dialogue on this theme, which we hope will become more intensive over the coming months.

National inter-agency co-operation regarding nutrition in schools

Michel CHAULIAC[1], Directorate General of Health, Paris, France

This paper provides a revealing insight into policy development at a national level in relation to the promotion of healthy eating in schools.

It is recognised that, as well as a biological function, food has economic, social and cultural dimensions. Its study involves many scientific disciplines. The need for action involving many sectors in order to ensure the protection and promotion of good nutritional status is a leitmotiv found in every document on food and nutrition policies and on nutritional education, which is one of their tools. The function of schools is to educate, which means that they have a specific role, which goes beyond the compulsory syllabus: all children can benefit from early teaching and learning in a supervised environment, under the guidance of educational specialists. Thus many people would like to make use of schools, particularly those who wish to promote greater well-being in society. One example is provided by the health sector. In the face of risks, and in a desire to prevent them, there is heavy demand for the inclusion in syllabuses of issues relating to mental health, sexuality, the dangers of tobacco and alcohol, behaviour involving risk, road safety, nutrition, etc. Nutrition is a special case, for large numbers of children spend a lot of their day at school. They have a physiological requirement to take in food during this period.

What are the questions which arise with regard to school nutrition? It is necessary to identify these issues carefully in order to determine how inter-ministry or inter-institution co-operation can help to facilitate and reinforce action. Then a look will be taken at the practical form taken by this co-operation in France, through the national nutrition and health programme.

Schools and nutrition

Advancing knowledge in the fields of epidemiology, medical sciences and human sciences underlines the important role played by nutrition as a determining factor in the main pathologies which impose the heaviest burden in terms of mortality and morbidity in Europe. In fact, it is during childhood, when eating habits are being formed, that the basis for such pathologies is created.

---

1. The opinions expressed in this part are the sole responsibility of the author.

An ever-present incentive to consume derives from changes in eating habits and in food supply and promotion, changes which result from the distance between home and workplace, family relationships, the ever-increasing availability and affordability of foodstuffs, the ease with which foods can be preserved and tailored more and more specifically to increasingly specific population groups. People's great concern about food safety has resulted in increased surveillance by the authorities. The regulations lay down strict criteria. Checks are carried out. Warning systems have been improved. The food chain, from producer to retailer and caterer, via the processor, has seen considerable progress. Now, food safety is regarded as an absolute requirement by the whole population. Consumers penalise severely any shortcomings in respect of safety. Where food safety is concerned, there can be no competition. So enjoyment and health are becoming factors in the competition in the food business. Nowadays, children, who are particularly fond of sweet products, determine what food the family buys.

The marked increase over the last two decades in the number of overweight and obese children has become a major concern of the health authorities. It is recognised that what is learnt during childhood influences the eating habits of the future adult. Children learn what is regarded as 'right' in the culture in which they live, and acquire the eating habits of the society in which they were born. However, neither what is 'right' nor habits are set in stone, but are continually changing. Consequently there can be no question of setting a rigid standard at a national, European or world level.

Nutrition at school: aims and strategies

The importance of beginning nutritional education in childhood is very widely accepted, so schools have a significant role to play, complementing that of the family. Two factors need to be clarified: the aim and how to attain it. Leaving aside specific interests, society, through the state, has to provide the answers.

It is important to promote, both individually and collectively, conduct beneficial to health, bearing in mind the fact that the nutritional environment is bound to undergo constant change. The purpose of this general guideline is to maintain, in the long-term, a good state of nutrition, a pre-requisite of a good state of health, and to prevent the development of pathologies.

School and the family are the two interactive environments for acquiring knowledge and learning about practice. They can direct the other influences to which children are subjected (the media and the promotional activity which filters into the family and school environments). It is therefore essential to foster convergence and consistency between the messages and practices transmitted at school, in the family and beyond that, in the social environment.

In a field in which individual and collective statements about food and its associations are as much about magic or beliefs as they are about science, this is a complex exercise. In 2000, French people, when questioned for a major food survey, made it clear that the messages were so contradictory that they did not trust anyone.

School food provision is varied in Europe and reflects the specific cultural history of each country. In order to promote eating habits beneficial to health, it is necessary for each country to clarify and make consistent the objectives set with regard to nutrition. The process should be carried out by the departments responsible for education, food, school health, and public health.

Nutrition at school: the French approach under the national nutrition and health programme

The school meals service

Each country has its own specific institutional system. In France, it is general practice for a full, hot lunch to be served in schools from kindergarten to upper secondary school. Parents can order meals if they wish for their children (aged from two to 12) from the primary school canteen, managed by the municipality. In secondary education, the provision of meals is a responsibility of the national education system, whereas the local or regional authorities are responsible for the premises – the departments, in the case of lower secondary, and the regions for upper secondary schools. The preparation of meals may be contracted out to a company.

Electorally, this service constitutes a major issue. The quality of the meals served at school is the subject of frequent debates involving children, parents, elected representatives and citizens. Menu committees are set up comprising councillors and parents' and schools' representatives, to discuss meal quality and other problems raised by school canteens. In 1998 during a general election campaign, at a time when unemployment was at record levels, a study showed that there had been a decrease in the numbers of lower secondary pupils in underprivileged areas eating in school canteens. Each political party made proposals to remedy the situation. Likewise, the wide-ranging debate resulting from the 'mad cow disease' crisis led those responsible for school canteens to ban beef on a temporary basis, under parental pressure. Beef did not reappear for a long time, returning when experts had given the go-ahead, and when guarantees of product origin could be both given and checked.

Other food provision in schools

At primary school, and especially in kindergartens, some municipalities may organise a snack outside school hours for children who have to await a parent's arrival after the end of the school day. Very often, at teachers' initiative, a snack is organised during the morning at kindergartens; this happens less frequently in primary schools. Parents are asked to bring food to be shared out. Under pressure from the children, and in view of the storage conditions, biscuits or sweet products predominate. In addition, some schools may qualify for free deliveries of milk.

Individual secondary schools often decide to install machines from which drinks, sweet or savoury products may be obtained. These belong to outside companies, and part of the profit is used at the school's own discretion, often being administered by a pupils' association.

Nutrition in the syllabus

Nutrition is not a separate subject on school syllabuses. Some aspects of nutrition are covered at various ages, from kindergarten to the end of secondary education. These come under various subjects: biology, science and environmental studies, economics and social sciences essentially, but they are also taken into account in physical education and sport. Food is also a subject, which spans different subjects and may be explored within the various teaching procedures which have been more recently implemented by the national education system: artistic and cultural projects, fact-finding excursions and supervised practical work.

The monitoring of pupils' health

School medicine comes under the national Education Ministry. Systematic examinations of pupils are scheduled throughout their school life, in particular with a view to monitoring growth. The data collected are analysed on an aggregate local or regional, or even national basis, although not yet to a sufficient degree.

Inter-sectoral work in the context of a national programme

In 2000, in the light of advances in scientific knowledge about the relationship between nutrition and health, as well as the country's epidemiological nutritional data and people's desire for consistency in the messages they receive about nutrition, the French Prime Minister asked the Health Minister to draw up and co-ordinate a national nutrition and health programme, working with other ministries.

This political request from the Prime Minister enabled the national nutrition and health programme (PNNS) to be drawn up, under the aegis of the Health Minister, with the Ministers for Agriculture, Education, Youth and Sport, Research, Consumer Affairs and the Interior. The programme, drawn up for the period 2001-2005, sets specific quantified objectives and directs a range of activities on the basis of several strategies. Together, they are intended to enable the general objective of "improving the health of the population as a whole by way of action on nutrition¹ to be achieved. In this overall vision where the aims set concern the population at large, and where nutrition is seen as a determining factor in health, the school environment is a fundamental vector, but not the only one of a policy which enables the overall consistency hitherto yet to be achieved. One of the aims is to associate the many players with a food-related role. Families, children, teachers, health professionals and the food chain from production to distribution and catering are all involved. The setting-up of the programme's strategic committee, chaired by the Health Minister, illustrates that desire for the programme to be co-ordinated inter-institutionally. Going beyond even the involvement of several ministries, practical effect has been given to the participation and involvement of other players indispensable to the achievement of the objectives. These include, for example, not only the local and regional authorities, which, as has been seen, are responsible for school meals, but also food manufacturers and consumers. Moreover, and a few concrete examples of this will be provided, the strategic committee sets up specific working groups to make proposals, some of them relating more specifically to the school environment. A national policy can be carried out only with the strong involvement of local players. The necessary organisation is planned and is being put into place.

These co-ordination procedures have made possible a number of achievements.

Tangible achievements

School meals

In June 2001, the Minister of Education published a circular promised in the context of the PNNS. That circular,² 'on the composition of meals served in school canteens and food safety', was jointly signed by eight Ministers and State Secretaries.³ It was addressed to all managers in the national education system

---

1. Available in French on www.sante.gouv.fr; click on 'nutrition' in accès simplifié par thème for access to both the French and the English version
2. available at www.education.gouv.fr/bo/2001/special
3. Education, Economic Affairs and Finance, Agriculture, Labour and Solidarity, Interior, Health, Vocational Education and Consumer Affairs.

involved in the taking of decisions relating to school meals. Only such a wide-ranging consultation between ministries could enable every structure to be reached, in view of the diversity of actors involved in school meals. The circular is a result of the collaboration between ministries, nutrition experts and professionals, particularly in the field of catering, and parents of schoolchildren. It also benefited from the work carried out earlier by the National Food Council. It sets out the major changes necessary in terms of the nutritional composition of the meals served: fewer fats and more iron, calcium and fibres, fruit and vegetables. It also stresses the benefits of bread. It gives a variety of pointers, relating both to the environment in which children eat their meals and the time, which should be allowed for them to do so. It also emphasises the educational dimension of school meals, in terms of both the discovery of tastes and nutritional education, and stresses the pleasurable aspect of food. It gives very practical and precise information with a view to achieving variety over sequences of 20 meals, together with indications of portion size, depending on the child's age (see details in Appendix). It warns against the addition of salt and advocates water rather than sugary drinks. The circular provides details of snacks in order to limit their potential adverse impact in terms of children over-eating (complementary work is under way on this specific point). It lists and clarifies the rules designed to guarantee food safety and traceability. In 2004, the Ministry of Education plans to carry out a full evaluation of the impact of the circular.

Catering for children who suffer from food allergies

An inter-ministerial circular[1] signed by five ministers[2] and published in September 2003 reinforces and supplements earlier instruments designed, in particular, to enable children suffering from food allergies to benefit from the school meals service, and more generally from any meals which children take together. To this end, a document (the individually-tailored plan, known as the PAI) is drawn up jointly by the head of the school, the school doctor - in liaison with the family doctor - the parents and, ideally, the manager of the school canteen. This text suggests different approaches to preventing the exclusion of the child from meals taken together at school. In particular, it lays down conditions enabling the child to bring in a packed lunch.

---

1. available at www.education.gouv.fr/bo/2003/34
2. Interior, Internal Security and Local Freedoms; Youth, Education and Research; Health, Family and Disabled Persons; Agriculture, Food, Fisheries and Rural Affairs; delegate for school education and delegate for the family.

In France there was a total of 7,482 PAIs for food allergies in 2002, i.e. an average of one PAI for every 1,538 children. More than 71% of PAIs are for children in primary schools and kindergartens.

Nutrition and school lessons

Under the auspices of the PNNS strategic committee, a working group held meetings over a one-year period in order to make proposals for the integration of the nutritional dimension into school lessons. The group included not only representatives of the Ministries of Health, Youth and Sport and Education, but also representatives of agencies responsible for health education and food safety, parent-teacher associations, consumer organisations and associations of teachers, school doctors, sociologists and paediatricians.

The work carried out has brought to light the weaknesses in the present situation – notably the dispersal of knowledge between different subjects and across different levels, the weak link between theoretical knowledge and what is actually served up at mealtimes and the divergence between highly processed food and its presentation as coming from small-scale farm producers. Emphasis has been placed on all the possibilities, illustrated by numerous initiatives taken at particular establishments or by local education authorities. Proposals were submitted to the ministers in the last quarter of 2003.

Consistency of the 'messages' which relate to nutrition

As part of the PNNS, a food guide for everyone entitled 'Eat your way to health' was published in 2002 and widely distributed to the public. On the basis of the objectives set by the programme, this enabled eating guidelines to be defined and made known to French people. The programme provides for the guide to be tailored to suit specific target groups, particularly children and adolescents. Work on the document for children started in the last quarter of 2002, following the same procedure used for the guide for the general public.

Once the document has been published, there will be an advertising campaign, and it will be put on sale. It will subsequently be distributed free of charge through a number of different networks. Publication is scheduled for September 2004. On the basis of the initial work, the decision has been taken to write a guide for parents of children from birth to 18 years of age, and to publish a version specifically for adolescents.

Monitoring children's growth

Another example of this co-operation is the design, publication and distribution of tools designed to assist with the monitoring of individuals' state of nutrition. Body-mass index is a valuable indicator for diagnosing and monitoring nutritional status, particularly the risks of excessive body weight and obesity. It can also help to predict changes in children's nutritional status. Disks have been prepared by specialists. Booklets have been written to help doctors to interpret and channel their discussions with their patients. The children's disks have been widely distributed to health professionals, particularly paediatricians and school doctors, so that a wide range of children can be diagnosed and then, if need be, guided at an early stage from the school medical service towards health service treatment.

The local level and the multi-sectoral approach

The programme was launched in early 2001. The working method adopted, the broad approach to nutrition outside the confines of the health care sector (regarding both the membership of the strategic committee and the procedure used to draw up specific tools or recommendations) is appropriate to French people's increasing concern about food and nutrition matters. Institutionally, the efforts are taken further through the setting up of active multi-sectoral committees at regional level.

Experiments are being conducted to introduce fruit vending machines in secondary schools, which could, in the long run, replace vending machines dispensing sweet and savoury products, which ought not to be eaten to excess. In many establishments, specific efforts have been made to encourage children to discover new tastes and to appreciate fruit and vegetables as part of their school meals, thanks to supporting efforts by teachers and the active participation by school cooks. In some primary schools, the free distribution of fruit is intended to lead to an increase in fruit consumption both at school and in the family. In other schools, teaching tools have been developed with the support of health professionals and women's organisations with the intention of engaging children's critical faculties in the face of food advertising on television. An effort is also made to involve families in this process. In other places, networks for the prevention of obesity in children and adolescents are being tried out. A close link is provided between school doctors, local practitioners, hospitals and outside players, such as leisure centres and sports clubs.

Conclusion

Action in favour of nutrition goes beyond the strict sphere covered by education and health. The co-ordination of the PNSS, which the Prime Minister entrusted to the Health Minister, gives the authorities concerned the possibility of working together to achieve specific, quantified and measurable targets.

Within the bodies and the working groups created under the PNNS, which include representatives of ministries, business, NGOs and scientists, the possible synergies between the spheres of activity of each are investigated and steered by the objectives of the national policy. Channels of communication are organised at the regional level, enabling changes to be made to suit specific contexts. Thus efforts are directed towards maintaining overall consistency in the aim of the activities and the messages conveyed to the population as a whole (adults and children). It is essential that the gap between the knowledge imparted at school and eating habits, both at school and at home, is reduced to the minimum. This will help to establish eating habits that are entrenched in the national and regional culture, and capable of coping with the various constraints encountered in daily life and the rapid development of the products on offer, which are the subject of major advertising drives. The challenge is obviously a huge one. Practical advances have begun. As well as activities carried out at national level, we are witnessing a burgeoning of local initiatives carried out through partnership. Schools often play a key role. Evaluation is an important tool for carrying forward inter-sectoral discussion so as better to shape the action to be taken. It is still necessary to clarify the interrelationships between nutrition and food policies, in order to reinforce measures designed to guide the supply of food in a direction beneficial to the health of schoolchildren and their families.

Bibliography

Haut Comité de la Santé Publique. *"Pour une politique nutritionnelle de santé publique en France. Enjeux et propositions"* (For a public health nutrition policy in France. Challenges and proposals). Ed ENSP, Rennes 2000. 275 pp.

Mission d'animation des agrobiosciences. *"Etats Généraux de l'alimentation: que voulons-nous manger?" (What do we want to eat?)*. INRA Toulouse 2001.

Ministry for Labour and Solidarity. Decree of 31 May 2001 establishing a strategic committee of the national nutrition and health programme J.O. (Official Gazette) No. 137, 15 June 2001.

Council Resolution of 14 December 2000 on health and nutrition. Official Journal of the European Communities C 20/01.

World Health Organization: First Action Plan for Food and Nutrition Policy (WHO Regional Committee for Europe, 2000-2005). WHO Copenhagen, 2001, 46 pp.

Ministry for Education Circular No 2003-135, of 8 September 2003, on the taking into collective care of children and adolescents suffering from long-term health problems.

Ministry for Education Circular No 2001-118, of 25 June 2001, on the composition of meals served in school canteens and food safety.

INSERM, Collective expert assessment of obesity: its diagnosis and prevention in children. INSERM, Paris, 2000.

INSERM, Operational expert assessment of children's and adolescents' health and proposed ways of preserving it. INSERM, Paris, 2003, 190pp.

Ministry for Health, Ministry for Agriculture, health insurance system, INPES, AFSSA, InVS. *"La santé vient en mangeant: le guide alimentaire pour tous" (Eat your way to health: a food guide for everyone)*. 2002, 127 pp.

Ministry for Health, Ministry for Agriculture, health insurance system, INPES, AFSSA, InVS. *"La santé vient en mangeant: document d'accompagnement du guide alimentaire pour tous" (Eat your way to health: a companion to the food guide for everyone)*, intended for health professionals. 2002, 93 pp.

Fischler C. *"Alimentation, morale et société" (Food, morality and society)*, in Giachetti I Ed Identités des mangeurs, Image des aliments. CNERNA-CNRS, Paris, 1996, coll Polytechnica, 54 pp.

Chiva M, Mischlich D. *"Du bon usage des sens dans l'alimentation"* (Using our senses wisely in relation to food). In "Education nutritionnelle: équilibres à la carte", Baudier F, Barthélémy L, Michaud C, Legrand L ed , Paris, CFES, 1995, pp 27-43.

Fischler C. *"L'Homnivore"*. Paris, Odile Jacob, 1990.

Poulain JP. *"Manger aujourd'hui. Attitudes, normes et pratiques"* (Eating today. Attitudes, standards and practice). Toulouse, Privat, 2002.

Ministry for Employment and Health, Directorate General for Health. National nutrition and health programme (PNNS), 2001-2005. Cah. Nutr.Diét. 2001, 36: 207-216.

Appendix
Extract from the circular on the composition of foods served in school canteens and food safety

In order to help those responsible for catering to comply with nutritional recommendations, the appendix to the circular provides indications as to the serving frequency of the foodstuffs listed in the GPEMDA (for instance, the frequency of the inclusion of chips or other fried foods with a high fat content on the menu is limited, whereas the inclusion of cheeses and dairy products with a high calcium content is encouraged).

The circular specifies that menus must be drawn up so as to suit children's tastes as far as is possible, in order to ensure that meals are actually eaten.

Foodstuff serving frequency (GPEMDA)

FREQUENCY CHECK LIST

Period from ... to ... (at least 20 meals)	Starter	Protein-based dish	Vege-table	Dairy product	Dessert	Frequency observed	Recommended frequency
Starters >= 15% fat						/20	8/20 maximum
Products for frying and pre-fried products >= 15% fat						/20	6/20 maximum
Fresh or dried pastries >= 15% fat						/20	4/20 maximum
Protein-based dishes with protein: lipid ratio =<1						/20	2/20 maximum
Raw vegetables fruit						/20	15/20 minior
Individual or mixed vegetables other than dried (50% minimum)						/20	10/20
Dried vegetables, starchy foods or cereals						/20	10/20

Dishes based on fish >= 70% fish and protein: lipid ratio >= 2					/20	4/20 minimum
Red meat					/20	4/20 minimum
Dishes based on meat or reconstituted fish < 70% raw material of animal origin					/20	4/20 maximum
Cheeses or other dairy products >= 150 mg calcium					/20	10/20 minimum
Cheeses or other dairy products <150 mg calcium and >= 100 mg calcium					/20	8/20 minimum

Weights of portions of dairy products currently used in collective catering:

Yoghurt: 125 g
Fromage frais: 100 g
Cream desserts, baked custard, baked-custard-style jellied milk, other jellied milk desserts: 80 to 125 g
Mousses: 50 g
Matured cheeses: 30 g
Processed cheeses: 20 g

CALCIUM PER PORTION	TYPES OF DAIRY PRODUCT
Calcium > 300 mg per portion	Emmental and cooked pressed cheeses of the Comté type
Calcium < 300 and > 200 mg per portion	Blue Saint-Paulin and other pressed cheeses of the Cantal type Pressed cheese specialities
Calcium < 200 and > 150 mg per portion	Plain yoghurt Fruit yoghurt Roquefort cheese Saint-Nectaire cheese Raclette cheese Creamy desserts
Calcium < 150 and > 100 mg per portion	Camembert and soft cheeses with a mixed rind (Brie, Carré...) Tomme cheese Fromage frais Munster cheese Processed cheese Fruit yoghurt Flavoured yoghurt Cream desserts and crème caramel Rice or semolina mould Rice or semolina pudding Baked custard Fruit baked in batter (Clafoutis) Jellied milk desserts Soft cheese specialities
Calcium < 100 mg per portion	Fresh, dry and semi-dry goat's cheese Goat's cheese, petit suisse Processed cheese Speciality products based on fromage frais or blue cheese, mousses Rice pudding, semolina pudding, crème caramel Cream desserts Fromage frais Custard Fruit baked in batter (Clafoutis) Baked custard

Discussion: Partnerships for healthy choices

There was time only for a brief discussion led by the facilitator, Cristine Deliens, at the end of this session.

On the subject of milk provision in schools.......

Ulla Marja Urho (Finland). I was disappointed that there has not been any discussion about the importance of milk provision in schools at the forum.

Jeltje Snell (Netherlands). Perhaps because it is not that important an issue nutritionally. Lack of calcium in primary school children is not a problem in western Europe.

On the subject of commissioning work and partnerships......

Mark Karaczun (England). In the National Health Service in the UK we often divide issues on traditional clinical lines and lifestyle issues such as healthy eating cut across these. Therefore it may be that many commissioning or budget headings have to be addressed. We have to rebuild or remake the cake.

On the subject of parents, partnerships and school nutrition action groups (SNAGS)......

Gillian Kynoch (Scotland). SNAGS played an important role in Scotland in sharing a common disappointment about school meals provision and in sharing a vision about where they might go. Councils then took an interest and these local or regional initiatives created a pressure on government nationally.

On the subject of Young Minds shared vision.......

The Young Minds team stated that continuous access during the school day to free fruit and water for students of all ages was important. In addition they did not believe that 'junk food' should be banned but that healthy food should be less expensive. A pleasant dining environment was also seen as important.

Aileen Robertson (WHO) asked the Young Minds team how vegetables could be made more accessible to young people at school? Friso Annema in Young Minds answered that in The Netherlands vegetables were not available in school and that vegetables were perceived as something to eat after school at home.

Twenty-five poster papers were developed and exhibited by representatives from thirteen countries and these provided a rich source of information and a stimulus for informal debate at the forum.

Grouping and classifying such a diverse range of papers could have been done in many ways, however the following broad themes emerged from the fine detail of the submissions.

- Policy reviews
- Partnerships
- Education and training
- Utilising research
- Changing traditions
- The environment and sustainability

In this brief review, the submitting country and the number of the poster are given, which will allow the reader to refer to Appendix 2 and/or the forum proceedings for the full reference and further details if this is desired.

Policy reviews

Some posters reviewed the **policy infrastructure** in their respective countries or in other cases, described reviews of current situations, which are leading to **policy change**. In Wales (Poster 4), The Welsh Assembly Government and Food Standards Agency Wales (FSA) are working together with local partners to support a range of initiatives designed to influence nutrition and improve the food and drink available in schools.

The Welsh Network of Healthy School Schemes (WNHSS) provides a national policy framework for local schemes. 599 schools are currently participating and guidance has been issued on:

- nutritional standards for school lunches, which underpins legislation;
- the need for a whole school approach;
- the place of food in the school curriculum.

Other relevant initiatives involve 'The Heartbeat Award for Schools', which rewards those offering a co-ordinated approach to food safety, nutrition teaching and healthy options. In addition The Welsh Assembly/FSA's nutrition strategy, 'Food and Well-Being', lists children and young people as a priority group.

There has been an increase in local, healthy school schemes and individual schools have worked on nutrition issues such as healthy packed lunches as a school meal option and healthy drink vending. There has been an increase in fruit tuck shops in Welsh schools. Nationally, free milk is available, and water coolers and free breakfasts are being introduced to schools in disadvantaged areas. It appears that national policy and support is stimulating action at a local level.

A major policy initiative is underway in England (Poster 5) under the umbrella of 'The Food in Schools Programme'. This is a joint venture of the Department of Health and Department for Education and Skills to help address concerns around children's diets in England. The Department of Health strand comprises eight projects, which in principle follow the child through the school day. These are:

• healthier breakfast clubs;

• healthier tuck shops;

• healthier vending machines;

• water provision;

• dining room environment;

• healthier lunch boxes;

• cookery clubs;

• growing clubs.

Each initiative will focus on how best to embed such interventions into schools to gain maximum benefit, overcome barriers, address sustainability, funding/resource issues and ease of implementation. Final evaluation reports are due in October 2004 and the programme aims to disseminate best practice in a 'whole school approach' to enable schools to develop sustainable in-house strategies for improving the nutrition and diet of children. A multifaceted dissemination strategy will be developed, as no one approach is appropriate for all schools. Partnerships are considered integral to the sustainability of the programme in England.

Several posters involved reviews of what young people are eating with a goal of informing future policy developments. In Finland (Poster 12) a survey was undertaken with the aim of determining the school meal patterns of Finnish pupils from the 7th to 9th grade, to analyse the differences in relation to recommendations on school lunches. In 2003 over 3,000 pupils in 12 different schools located around the country, answered a structured questionnaire after the lunch break in classrooms. This survey had also been carried out in the years 1988, 1994, 1998 at the same schools. The results indicated that:

- 89% of pupils visited the school canteen;
- 95% of pupils ate the main course (this is more than on previous studies);
- 50% of pupils drank milk and 47% ate the salad (these are less than on previous studies);
- 60% of pupils liked the main dish;
- 60% of pupils used less than 10 minutes to eat the lunch;
- only 13% of pupils ate the planned meal with a warm dish, salad, milk and bread (this is less than before);

The study concluded that skipping school meals appears not to be common among Finnish pupils, but only a few of them eat a varied, balanced lunch. There are differences between boys and girls lunch models: boys more often eat the main course and drink milk, girls more often eat the salad and bread. The pupils see the planned lunch as an opportunity to make their own choices. Pupils more often drink milk when there are at least two types of milk (0% and 1.5% of fat) served. It was concluded that there are big differences between the school lunches offered in different schools although national guidelines exist in Finland. Making the guidelines mandatory and adding alternatives in salad, milk and bread are considered possible ways to improve the situation. It is also suggested that active follow-up and training of the canteen personnel will be important.

In Bulgaria (Poster 13) a national nutrition survey on over 7,000 schoolchildren aged 7 to 19 years was conducted. Nutrition was assessed using 24-hours recall and the food frequency method. Weight and height of schoolchildren were measured and information on physical activity, cigarette smoking habits and socio-economic characteristics of households were also collected.

Mean daily energy intakes for most age/gender groups were higher than the recommendations. Risk for inadequate energy input was observed for boys aged 10-14 corresponding to higher prevalence of underweight among them (6.8% with urban, 8.9% with rural residence). No risk for inadequate protein intakes was determined. Total fat consumed was 34.6-38%, SFA provided 11.3-12.7%. Mean daily intakes of calcium, iron, vitamin A, thiamin, riboflavin and folate were below RNI for all population groups (41.8-94% RNI). Physical activity of adolescents was low, corresponding to the high overweight prevalence, 23.3 % for boys, 19% for girls.

The obtained results were a basis for the development of a national programme for nutrition improvement of schoolchildren. A governmental policy for the improvement of schoolchildren's nutrition through school canteens and refreshment bars was published and is being implemented in Bulgaria.

In the Netherlands (Poster 22) there is a policy of promoting the consumption of fruit and vegetables in schools and a national three year programme for primary schools started in 2002, funded by the government and producers. The aim of the project is to encourage children to eat more fruit and vegetables each day, and the initiative also aims to raise awareness of fruit and vegetable intake and increase knowledge of recommendations.

Fruit and vegetables are distributed free of charge twice weekly to all grades of participating schools (now 276 in seven cities, aiming at 1,000 in 25 cities). In October 2003 educational materials were distributed (a teacher's guide, 26 lesson activities, parent leaflet, poster, five video films for 9 to 12 year olds, website, information service for schools, fact sheets and Q&A letters for intermediaries). Throughout the project, monitoring is done through collection of food consumption data: a baseline survey in experimental schools and control schools in The Hague and Almelo. The children will be followed in two other survey groups and process evaluation will also be undertaken. Effects will be measured in fruit and vegetable consumption and in the knowledge and attitudes of the children. This study will be completed in 2005.

Partnerships

The theme of **partnership working** is consistent with the health promoting school or whole school approach, and there was evidence of this approach in many of the posters submitted. An intervention in Portugal (Poster 1) is based on a model which recognises the importance of involving the pupils and teachers in the development of a cross-disciplinary classroom curriculum and also the need to involve a wider group of staff and parents as well as to take account of environmental factors.

The programme was conceived as a whole school approach to nutrition education with a theoretical basis on social learning theory. The target group was a school community (831 students/parents, 85 teachers, and 10 staff members of the catering sector).

The effectiveness of the intervention was determined using a pre- and post-test design using the retrospective 24 hours recall and food frequency methods; it was applied before and after a one-year intervention to 215 students (two classrooms of each level, from 5th to 9th grade). Opinion questionnaires before and after the programme development were also applied.

An improvement in the quality of meals made by students was detectable after the intervention, with differences according to the development level and gender.

Taste and food availability were set as determining factors influencing food consumption. It is concluded that a holistic approach to nutrition education is recommended which should involve all the partners in the educational process and that it should be developed over a longer time period, starting in the primary school.

A study from Spain (Poster 9) focused on the contribution of school meals to eating patterns of the school-aged population and evaluated the perceived quality of the service. The design of this research fully acknowledged the importance of the home/school partnership in influencing young people's food consumption.

A descriptive cross-sectional study was carried out on a random population sample (3 to 16 years) having school meals in Spain. The study protocol included socio-economic data, food consumption and dietary habits in the school and outside school. Information was collected by means of two questionnaires: one completed by children at school and a second one completed by the family at home.

The results indicated that lunch was a full meal for 90% of children. 70% of children perceived the portion served to be of adequate size. However, 55% of boys and 40% of girls aged 12-16 years reported eating only half the serving. Main reasons were dislike for taste (50%) and inadequate temperature (10%). In the school menu vegetables and fish were offered less frequently than other food groups. 45% had a mid-morning snack and 81% an after-school snack. The overall food consumption pattern showed an inadequate intake of fruit and vegetables.

The authors conclude that the results of the study provide interesting data on school meals in Spain. It is suggested that catering companies supplying the service could contribute to increase the offer of fruit and vegetables in schools, including a choice of a mid-morning and/or after-school snack particularly for children under 12 years.

In France (poster 11) a community partnership approach is being taken to support children in acquiring healthier eating habits. At the same time they are being given greater freedom to choose and to learn to make healthy food choices of their own. This is a two-year experimental project using a community-health approach that involves children, parents, professionals (teachers, caterers, school health staff) and the local council. The initiative took stock of the situation by listening to children and parents' concerns about quality of school life. Needs were identified, resources assessed, and action priorities and evaluation criteria agreed upon taking account of local priorities.

The objectives agreed with the school community were to:

- offer balanced canteen meals that children would actually eat;
- encourage children to try unfamiliar dishes at tasting sessions;
- cut down on snacking during the day;
- promote eating of fruit and vegetables and reduce consumption of high calory foods;
- encourage children to build physical exercise into their daily routine.

After one school year:

- the school community was enthusiastic about the project;
- there was evidence of changes in eating habits (less afternoon snacking, more balanced meal choices);
- canteen staff requested training in food education;
- tasting sessions introduced the children to new foods.

The next stage of the project will look at these issues in the context of related lifestyle issues such as the promotion of physical exercise and it will include measures such as body mass index as a biological indicator in relation to obesity.

The French-speaking community in Belgium (Poster 15) has been supporting health promotion schemes to improve meals in elementary and primary schools since 1996. A forum was organised in December 2000 under the joint initiatives of the Ministries of Health and Education allowing consultation between schools, health professionals, caterers, parents as well as local authorities. 'Cordes', a non profit organisation financed by the government of the French-speaking community of Belgium co-ordinates these projects – 'A table les cartables' and 'Midis à l'école' and is in charge of counselling schools and partners.

A health promoting school approach is taken to enhance the capacity of in-school actors and other partners to develop joint 'healthy eating' projects. Meal organisation (packed lunches and hot meals) varies greatly from one school to another. Each school is thus encouraged to develop a health-promoting project adjusted to the local needs expressed by pupils and their teachers. The process gives children the opportunity of acknowledging school priorities as well as those of the persons in charge of meals. Teachers are given support through counselling and tools, thus leading to a participatory approach. Educational leaflets are made available systematically to involve parents, caterers, school health professionals and local authorities. Each school council is invited to adopt a charter for healthy eating at school and to organise discussion on priorities. The educational approach is focusing on choice and the theme of 'healthy eating' is approached through side issues to raise children's interests: how food is produced, what are the bodily needs and health requirements, eating with our senses, etc. Children are involved in the design and development of the project at classroom or school level. The different points of view makes them aware of the process of collective decision-making and outcomes.

According to an ongoing survey, more than half of the schools in the French-speaking part of the country have put better lunchtimes (meals and playtimes) among their priorities for change. A diversity of solutions has come out of the consultation process. The pupils' contributions showed considerable ingenuity and originality; the health implications of nutrition are better known; the large and renewed distribution of tools for teachers, parents, health actors and school staff has helped to fuel discussion.

Developing joint projects as a result of a consultation process obviously requires time and continuous support for participants. Rather than prescribe ideal eating habits, the aim is to stimulate pupils' curiosity, a desire to participate and the ability to make the right choices for better health. The relationship between a democratic process in schools and health promotion is made evident. The participation of the pupils themselves, their families and those responsible for producing school meals calls into question the traditional decision-making process and school management methods. It is suggested that external resources from the community, the health sector or from different stakeholders (food industry and distribution, caterers, families, politicians) should be able to focus on the healthy choice target rather than on the interests of a specific sector.

In Denmark (Poster 18) there is a growing awareness of the fact that partnerships between different stakeholders can be a powerful tool in the promotion of healthy lifestyles. Stakeholders include authorities, practitioners, researchers, NGOs and private enterprises. The advantage is that through partnerships it is possible to obtain much greater effect of campaigns and policy implementations than stakeholders can obtain through individual efforts. This paper explores the Danish experience in a public NGO partnership project that aims at developing healthy school meal catering systems in Danish municipalities.

The paper evaluates the experiences from the project 'Meals for children in day care and schools.' It asks the questions: what are the characteristics of partnerships in this context? What are the perspectives of NGOs and authorities working together? What are the limitations? Can other stakeholders be involved and what are the further obstacles in developing healthy school meal catering in Denmark?

The project was carried out in co-operation with the Danish research institute for Food Safety and Nutrition and the Danish Dietetic Association. The project aimed at carrying out an information campaign on healthy school meal catering targeted at the important stakeholders in and around the school environment. In Denmark provision of school meals is not compulsory and hence it is up to the municipalities and schools to decide whether school meal catering is to be provided. In most cases no school meal catering exists and food is mostly provided by parents by means of an ordinary lunch box. However the idea of public provision of school meals enjoys support from parents and from many politicians. The reason is that unhealthy eating habits can be influenced in this way and also busy parents have the possibility of avoiding preparing a lunch box. As a result many schools are open to the idea that school meals should be provided.

The project consisted of three parts. An explorative research part based on a multiple qualitative case study in a number of schools and institutions aimed at identifying obstacles and barriers towards healthy eating, preparation of a handbook aimed at issuing guidelines to overcome these obstacles and barriers and a dissemination part aimed at making the result available for the food and professionals in schools and institutions.

Based on these findings a handbook on meals in daycare centres and schools was published. The handbook (Christensen et al, 2002) contains guidelines for developing healthy school meal systems and is targeted towards the different actors in the school and institution environment who are involved in meal provision. The release of the handbook was accompanied by papers in professional journals and were announced on the 'Diet in a nutshell' website (www.altomkost.dk). In addition a series of meetings with practitioners was held.

This poster discusses the outcome of the campaign measured in terms of penetration of the material and in particular the advantages and disadvantages in carrying out campaigns in cooperation between a public authority and a NGO.

In the Netherlands (Poster 23) a collaborative approach to health promotion in schools entitled Schoolbeat uses a co-ordinated approach, including parental and student participation and attempts to expand school health into the surrounding community areas of the school.

In this partnership regional health promoting agencies with a focus on mental health, addiction, public health, social welfare and individual student care have joined forces. The aim is to work via new health promoting school teams, assisted by one of the workers of the collaborating agencies. These teams consist ideally of the school care-co-ordinator, a parent, a student and a prevention worker. The prevention worker is trained to represent all the collaborating agencies and to assist the teams in choosing health promotion activities based on school health data and input from parents, teachers and students. A Schoolbeat quality-checklist is developed to gain insight into the quality and effectiveness of school health promotion programmes, including programmes promoting healthy eating.

Schools are experiencing many difficulties in developing adequate provision for problem students. As a result they are, at the moment, less interested in investing in health promotion. To ensure successful tailored school health promotion a chain-care approach is under development linking school health promotion with individual pupil care.

Education and training

A group of papers either had a strong focus on **classroom education** or they explored issues relating more broadly to the **education and training** of a wider group of participants including the teachers.

One education initiative was developed in Portugal (Poster 2) with the aim of increasing knowledge and of improving eating practices of school children enrolled in two basic schools. The sample included 102 children, aged 9 to 13. Children's food habits were assessed with two 24h-recall, one before the intervention and the other six weeks after its end. Knowledge acquisition was assessed with a questionnaire, in which children were asked to name healthy foods and to give their definition of healthy food habits. The programme was designed to reach the school community and several educational materials were developed.

The results showed an increase in the number of meals per day and also in the food quality index. Knowledge acquisition was also observed as the number of students answering increased and also the contents of the answers improved. These outcomes reveal that these two broad objectives were achieved with a simple but effective programme.

Another development in Portugal (Poster 3) 'Discover healthy eating' is an interactive CD-ROM for schoolchildren, aged 11–14. This educational material was developed by the Faculty of Nutrition and Food Sciences from the University of Porto in collaboration with the Consumer Institute and financed by Health Programme XXI.

The objectives of the CD-ROM are to facilitate the transmission of information and to improve knowledge and understanding in the area of food and nutrition sciences, to stimulate co-ordinated work among students, teachers and family as well as to help youngsters to adopt healthy eating behaviours and to practise physical activity regularly.

The design and graphics of the CD are centred around a fridge which displays on the door several magnets, each one corresponding to a different section: an interactive video, games, knowledge tests, library and a competition. The interactive video represents one day in the life of a young boy during which he goes to school, plays, eats and does some household tasks. The player can interact by making different food choices which will affect the boy's activities.

The games, tests and library, which are connected with food and nutrition, are intended to bring together learning and fun. Finally, the national competition entitled 'The Dish of My Region' involves the filling in of one questionnaire by a student and then a culinary preparation of his/her region taking into account healthy nutrition, sustainability, environmental and cultural aspects.

In England, The Food Standards Agency funds research (Poster 6) into the major barriers consumers face to making healthier dietary choices and evaluation of interventions to help overcome these barriers.

Two evaluated school-based interventions were undertaken:

- Bash Street Kids. A whole school approach, for one school year, to encourage increased fruit and vegetable intake in children aged six to seven and 10 to 11 in England. The fruit and vegetable intake of pupils in two test and two control schools in Scotland was assessed by food diaries at baseline and post-intervention.

- Dish it Up! An interactive CD-ROM. Background research with, and active involvement of, the target age group of pupils aged 11 and 12 was used to develop a motivational CD-ROM. This includes fun and challenging quizzes and games related to food choices and provides a visual assessment and feedback of the teenager's diet. It was briefly evaluated after use in lessons in a number of UK schools.

There was a small but significantly higher average consumption of 0.5 portions of fruit per child per day in intervention schools compared with control schools.

Teacher support material featuring the Bash Street cartoon characters is being adapted for the Food Standards Agency website. In addition there was a significant improvement in pupils' knowledge, but no change in attitude or behaviour as a result of short exposure to the CD-ROM. The Agency has provided three free copies of the CD to every secondary school in the UK.

The research tends to confirm the effectiveness of an integrated approach and the difficulties with a dietary assessment tool for this age group. It proved difficult to get parents involved and the heavy dependence on the researcher input may limit sustainability.

In Scotland, NHS Health Scotland and The Child and Adolescent Research Unit of the University of Edinburgh have developed a training resource (Poster 7) that explores the psycho-social aspects of healthy eating and provides current research findings in an accessible way. Healthy eating choices at school require the support of school staff who understand the complex issues relating to young people's eating choices both in school and in their wider lives. A case study approach to health promoting schools through healthy eating identified that there are many issues that impact on the choices young people make about food and that teachers wished more support with these complex issues. The resource is targeted at trainers who will be able to work with teachers and school health coordinators in the upper primary and lower secondary school. The resource includes nine background chapters in three sections. The titles of the chapters indicate the wide scope of the resource, these are:

- Growing & Changing - Food for Growth, Physical Activity, Adjusting to Puberty;

- Food & Young People - Food Patterns and Preferences, Overweight and Obesity, Dieting and Eating Disorders;

- Image and Reality - Self-esteem, Body Image, the Role of the Media.

The pack will include a set of eight fact sheets for the teachers and offer guidance on how to train teachers in relation to the issues identified in the chapters. The resource provides five training sessions that cover the above issues. These acknowledge the importance of starting with the learner's own agenda. The resource also gives trainers a menu of activities to use in training that are linked to the background chapters.

On completion of the development phase and testing, Health Scotland will publish the manual in 2004 and it will be made freely available to other European countries to use and adapt as they consider appropriate.

A project in Denmark (Poster 16) aims to support motivated schools in establishing healthy meals and other food options for the pupils. 'Diet in a nutshell – a taste for life' is a three year project initiated in October 2002 by the Danish Minister of Food, Agriculture and Fisheries and carried out by the Danish Veterinary and Food Administration. As of August 2003 regional offices have, as part of their job function, the responsibility to coach/guide and support local schools in the process of establishing healthy school meals and/or formulate nutritional policies in this field. The aim of the regional approach is to enhance the anchoring and empowerment processes of initiatives regarding meals in school. An educational programme to support employees has been established and evaluated.

Through an educational programme of 12 working days, 12 regional food specialists have been equipped to carry out the duty of guidance and support of schools. One of the aims of the programme has been to update their current knowledge in the field of nutrition. This has been undertaken through workshops which focus on a variety of issues e.g. 'Nutritional status of Danish children', 'Children's recommended intake of carbohydrates' and 'Focus on hygiene'. Furthermore, the aim of the programme has been to sharpen the participant's communicative skills and ability to coach/guide, which is vital for the success of this project.

The workshops aim to combine theory and practical assessments, focusing on, for example, 'How to plan and manage a meeting with different stakeholders' and 'How to coach in changing processes'.

The evaluation showed overall that 58% of the participants thought the content of the course was excellent and very relevant. 33% disagreed slightly as they were only satisfied with the course and 9% were not satisfied. The results show that the course participation has been impressive with a participation rate of 98%. This may be due to the candidate selection procedure and the attraction of undertaking this new task.

Due to their independent and isolated job function, it has been decided to establish a network of the regional employees. Therefore a national team has now been set up. The group meets once a month to exchange experiences regarding the development of partnerships locally, cross-culture collaboration, involvement of stakeholders and to gain new knowledge regarding healthy meals in schools. Furthermore the project co-ordinators will supervise the regional employees by phone and through visits in schools.

A project with some related features, such as the goal of developing skills at a local level, is being developed in The Netherlands (Poster 21). This three and a half year project promoting good cafeteria policies is aimed at four areas: the food offered; hygiene; integrating lessons and cafeteria practice; and written policy plans. The Netherlands Nutrition Centre cooperated with three regional health services to develop this approach. After situation analysis, project materials were developed and piloted in ten schools in 2001-2002. Action teams of school leaders, teachers, catering staff, 12-16 year old students and parents were supported by the project team during four visits. Three pilot schools used the materials without support. A process and effect evaluation was done using semi-structured interviews, written questionnaires and hygiene quick scans. The results indicated that:

- schools with committed school managers had better results;
- one school year is too short to create essential conditions for success (special budget, time for training, partnerships);
- schools found implementing hygiene norms impossible without training;
- the range of food offered could be balanced;
- students need more than lessons to actually buy the healthy choice;
- process facilitation is essential as pilot schools without support of the project team had not made much progress.

It is recommended that regional health services should take on facilitation but for technical advice other professionals are needed. National implementation started in September 2003 and this now involves the dissemination of pilot results, the adaptation of pilot materials for national use and the setting up of structures and training in national workshops.

Utilising research

The theme of **utilising existing data**, and the factors which influence **the use or under-use of research**, was explored in a group of papers.

A qualitative review from Belgium (Poster 14) provides an important context for all the research described in the posters and also for the research referred to in the main papers at the forum. The starting point of this study was the finding that information is under-utilised when projects are developed by those who play an active role in the field.

The general objective of the study was to identify those factors, which, positively or negatively, influence information use by persons with an active role in nutrition education for young people. This was done by setting up semi-directive discussions with ten persons with an active role in nutrition education, in or out of school, in the French speaking community of Belgium.

Half of those questioned said that they make use of youth obesity statistics. Information is used mainly during project preparation, and very little during evaluation. Respondents quote the following factors among the various elements, which influence data use:

- the visibility of information;
- shortage of time to search for information;
- lack of training in how to interpret information;
- a dearth of local data;
- a lack of clear interpretation of findings.

This study enabled elements fostering or curbing data use to be identified. Among the main problems that it highlighted are not so much lack of data, but lack of local data. The fact that the information available is used by few of those who have a direct role in the field is also evident.

In Denmark (Poster 20) a qualitative study looked at the practical and financial barriers, which can result in the failure of healthy eating projects. The project had two aims: 1) to investigate the barriers faced by schools and day-care centres and their consultancy needs when setting up meal provision schemes; and 2) to develop inspirational material providing knowledge to those implementing meal schemes, in order to facilitate the establishment of these.

Observations were made with leaders, teaching staff and kitchen personnel in three kindergartens and four schools with distinct meal provision schemes. The purpose was to discover the barriers and needs in a broad cross-section of distinct approaches to organising meal provision schemes. In the case of kindergartens, food was prepared internally in all three cases. In two of the kindergartens, children were involved in the preparation of meals as an educational element, and in two of the cases, special kitchen personnel were employed. In one case, a teacher was responsible for preparation. The study showed that tight finances and the organisation of practical matters are major barriers to the setting-up of meal provision schemes. In addition, the study also showed that deficient cooperation between professional groups and lack of support for meal provision initiatives constituted substantial barriers to efficient meal provision schemes. Poor and deficient knowledge of food safety and rules applicable in the area were also barriers for some.

Inspirational material has been prepared on the basis of the study, 'Food for Children in Day-care Centres and Schools' with advice on the following:

- getting started (a schedule);
- food and meal policies;
- choice of food and meal provision scheme (finances and practical organisation);
- the food and the meal;
- organic food;
- food hygiene.

It was concluded that knowledge about issues such as practical circumstances, finances and food safety is important when a meal provision scheme is to be set up, and inspirational material with specific directions is of great assistance to those implementing schemes. To support the initiatives and work with the various professional groups, written information is not always sufficient, and personal consultation and guidance is often necessary. The project has contributed to identifying some of the areas, in which a new travelling team (as described in Poster 16) will give advice on the establishment of meal provision schemes. This travelling team now uses the inspirational material in its consultancy services.

In the Basque country, Spain (Poster 10), a study was undertaken utilising the data available in the 'Monitoring programme of school meals in Bilbao'. Started in 1984, this programme has been co-ordinated by the Community Nutrition Unit and implemented in collaboration with the School Health and Food Safety Programmes. It collects information on key indicators, provides advice to caterers and school food service personnel and develops information materials for families and schools. Annual surveillance on a random sample of children considers food intake in the school (double weight food record of school meal) and out of school (24 hour recall) along with the perceived quality of the service. Organisational issues, management and satisfaction is collected from managers and food service staff.

Analysis of the data indicated that 7,753 students (3 to 16 year) and 203 teachers used the service in Public Schools of Bilbao (n=45), 172 students and six teachers per school on average in 2001-2002. Most schools were supplied by catering companies (81.8%); the rest prepared food on site. Special care services were supplied for 178 students with special needs. Food allergy, cerebral palsy, psychomotor problems, physical handicap, coeliac disease or special dietary requirements were main causes. School food service personnel scored highest for perceived quality, followed by educational and recreational activities linked to school meals. The lunchroom scored the lowest.

It is evident that the Bilbao school meal programme has significantly contributed to the provision of a school food service to meet the specific needs of students and schools. The programme highlights not only the nutritional quality of food supply, but also the educational dimension of school meals by providing students with the opportunity to develop and practice skills supportive of a healthy diet.

Changing traditions

This is a theme that was important in several papers, but was central to two projects in particular.

In the Netherlands (Poster 24) there is not a tradition of providing a hot meal in the middle of the day for school pupils. In fact 460,000 schoolchildren (almost 1/3 of the total) lunch daily at school with packed lunches brought from home. The Netherlands Primary School Act states that schools only need to provide a room for those children remaining at school during lunchtime. It is for parents to decide if school lunches should be provided or if supervision should be provided for packed lunch consumption.

The Association for Public Authority Education (Vereniging Voor Openbaar Onderwijs, -VOO) wants to promote good quality food provision in schools. In order to establish the need for providing hot meals at schools, a pilot in two schools with three locations in Almere was started. A caterer, Apetito, was hired to deliver meals four days a week, over a period of two weeks. Infrastructure was improved and the meals met the standards of the Netherlands Nutrition Centre with lunch supervisors trained to support the provision. During the pilot the meals were free of charge. All parents were informed of the initiative: 75 out of 100 wanted their child to participate. Parents were invited to attend a 'tasting' workshop; of the 45 parents enrolled, only 13 actually attended. 82 children completed a short questionnaire and participated in group interviews at the three locations. 68% of parents participating in the pilot completed the questionnaire. Parents could also debate the issue on the VOO website. The lunch supervisors were also interviewed.

Almost all pupils indicated that they liked the food; 72-84% thought the temperature of the food and the portion size was good and that they would like to eat at school every day. Children stated in the group interviews that they ate everything, which was often not the case at home.

Parents who attended the 'tasting' workshop were very positive about the meals, the quality was judged even more positively after the session. Some parents indicated they would like more salad served. Half of the responding parents thought the meals a good idea; they were positive about the quality of the meals, the portion size and the variety of the menu. They did not think serving hot meals at school would deteriorate the quality time parents want to spend with their children. When asked about the price they would be willing to pay for a hot meal for their children, half were willing to pay the indicated price of 3.25 euro per meal; others would rather pay less.

The lunch supervisors were positive about the pilot, especially about the positive reactions of the children. They found the pilot rather time intensive and wished for better equipped facilities in the school. On the basis of the pilot results, the VOO is now offering all public schools and kindergartens in the Netherlands the possibility to have hot meals catered.

In Germany (Poster 25) another traditional practice, that of half day schooling, is changing and this is providing an opportunity to consider the nutritional needs of the young people and the role of the education service in meeting these needs. In many schools there are no canteens and outside caterers will provide a service. Tender preparation is often carried out by persons with limited knowledge of all necessary aspects. These are wide-ranging from what constitutes healthy nutrition for children to what demands can be made of the catering sector.

Commissioned by the Senate Department of Education, Youth and Sport of Berlin together with the health insurance fund AOK, the organisation Organic Food Service Consultancy (ÖGS) defined the targets for appropriate school nutrition as encompassing the most up-to-date state of nutrition research as well as sustainability and economic principles. Dietary principles were adopted from guidelines of the Research Institute of Child Nutrition (FKE) and the German Nutrition Society (DGE e.V.).

A tender document was created considering all the above-mentioned aspects together with a key for the evaluation of tender submissions. The tender documents can be adapted according to a municipality's objectives. For example the amount of organic or regional produce to be included in the menu specifications can be adapted. Thus the public sector can play an important role in meeting key objectives on nutrition, environment and fair business practices.

The environment and sustainability

Healthy eating is about more than the biochemistry nutrition. The broad issues of the environment and sustainability were recurring themes especially in papers from Germany, Denmark, Sweden and The Netherlands.

The issue of healthy organic food was also a theme in two posters from Denmark. The first study (Poster 17) refers to the fact that, in Denmark, there is no tradition of young people having the opportunity to buy food at school. Instead Danish children bring a packed lunch from home. However studies have shown that 25% of the children in Copenhagen do not bring a packed lunch.

The Copenhagen Municipality has adopted a policy in which the Municipality takes responsibility for introducing healthy eating habits as well as for creating pleasant eating environments in schools. It is also a goal to create habits that children can benefit from in their adult life. In addition, the municipality wants to influence the social inequalities, which are associated with many health problems, through intervention in the school environment. It is the view of this project that an important part of healthy school food provision is to implement the goal that the municipality uses at least 75% of organic food in the public kitchens. The Copenhagen Municipality has the following nutritional goals for the period 2002-2005: More inhabitants should eat healthily. This aim is part of the plan for public health and has five strategic goals for public health in Copenhagen. The plan is divided into 13 areas for action and nutrition is one of them.

To reach this goal the Municipality wants to:

- prevent overweight by encouraging inhabitants at risk to lose weight;
- introduce healthy food and dietary habits among inhabitants;
- implement a nutrition policy for institutions in Copenhagen;
- introduce healthy and organic school food for children in schools.

In 2001 the Copenhagen Municipality decided to establish provision of school meals for the whole community. The project will implement adopted goals for nutrition in the Municipality and is in agreement with the Copenhagen Municipality policy concerning sustainability and use of organic foods. The criteria for success is "all 30,000 students in Copenhagen should be offered organic, healthy, affordable meals at school on a daily basis".

Through the school food project the municipality wants to focus on:

- education, learning, organic and health promotion through the development of physical and organisational tools that empower children;

- educating the students as health ambassadors by involving them in meal provision;
- in service training of teachers;
- co-operation between the kitchens in the Municipality and suppliers of organic products;
- establishing organic production facilities for the school meals;
- school milk provision in all schools;
- education in autocontrol programmes and hygiene.

There is an interaction between the students' health, well-being, learning capacity and eating habits. The availability of food and the social and physical area have a considerable impact on the children's food habits. By means of the project 'Copenhagen Organic Healthy School Food' the municipality supports the food habits of the schoolchildren. School food is not just a matter of offering more meals. School food has also an important educational component too. By educating the students and by influencing their attitudes and values in terms of food, healthy eating and environment it is possible to empower the students. The school has the opportunity to facilitate children's learning about healthy food in general and through this to prevent lifestyle and nutritional related diseases.

Another Danish project 'The Good Meal' (Det Gode Måltid) (Poster 19) also has an emphasis on organic food provision. It is part of an ongoing development and reorientation project in the municipality of Roskilde.

Roskilde regards food and meals as important parameters for quality and responsibility in the municipality. The objective for the municipality is to enlarge the choice of meals in the local institutions. It is a goal to provide 'The Good Meal' to all users of public institutions. The aim of the project is to solve the nutritional problems that inevitably exist in the municipal food chain. National investigations suggest that 1/3 of the senior citizens are undernourished, primarily because they do not eat enough. As for pupils and young people they also eat insufficiently in terms of both amount and nourishment. The municipality plans to reorientate public provision of meals into 100% organic grown food. The strategy is one of reorientation rather than one of conversion. By implementing a 'reorientation in minds and pots' we aim to secure a permanent change in purchases and food production. After the reorientation, the resources of the municipality will be economically as well as environmentally sustainable. The motto is that the public sector ought to be and can be a locomotive in the agricultural change-over to organic production.

In concrete terms, 'The Good Meal' consists of four independent food and meal initiatives for schools, nurseries, old age homes, and the construction of a new production unit 'Children`s Food', which will provide for the school canteens and the nurseries.

The projects have the following objectives, the fulfilment of which is our criteria for success:

- enhance public meal provision and thereby encourage the abolition of the packed lunch;
- make the eating environment more attractive and improve the culinary component of the meal;
- increase the ecological part of the raw materials as much as the economy allows. The goal is to reach 100% ecological meals;
- secure the recommended nutrition for the target group concerned;
- be constructive and critical regarding improvement of the existing food supply;
- secure an improvement of the quality of the existing meals in the municipality;
- make food culture an integrated part in the life of children and adults. Take initiatives to remove the barriers that hinder this development.

Our experience shows that most kitchens are able to introduce up to 100% organic food within the existing meal economy. However, a reorientation strategy requires changes in investments. An ecological reorientation, rather than conversion, is a growing process that creates changes in both meal preparation as well as in the eating environment.

A Swedish study (Poster 8) identified variations between schools and the strengths/weaknesses in the school-lunch system, such as:

- the composition of total meals;
- the time schedule for serving;
- the influence of dining room logistics and number of people in dining room on intake and waste;
- the influence of adult attendance on intake and waste;
- the participation in school lunches in different age groups of students;
- the menu preferences in different age groups.

The target groups for the study were local politicians and other decision makers responsible for school lunches.

During a two week period, all food served in the dining rooms, salads, main and side courses and other (left-over) courses was weighed before being served. Bread, drink and special food such as vegetarian or ethnic foods were not weighed. Leftover food was weighed on return to the kitchen, as well as all scrap waste from plates. A nutritionist calculated the recommended weight of the 20 meals, suitable for intake by a pupil of about 10-13 years of age.

A financial estimation of an average price for the main course was made to enable an estimate of the cost of waste and surplus production from the central kitchen to be established. The number of students whom the central kitchen, the schools, and the central administration included when invoicing, was collected and compared. The number of students and adults for whom food was ordered was noted. The number of people who came to eat was calculated by counting the plates used (including the plates used by those who had special food). Timetables for when lunch was served to the students were collected, as well as information on how many people were allowed, according to safety regulations, to be in the dining-room at the same time. Information about sales in, and opening hours of, school cafeterias during the two weeks was gathered. During the same six days, the kitchen staff filled in a form noting what they served as salads and side-courses to the main meal so that total meals offered in schools could be compared to national recommendations.

A systemic approach was vital so as to avoid the risk of seeking fault in any specific participants. A system is an indivisible whole. The result of the whole system is a consequence of the interaction between the results of the parts – not the sum of the result of the parts! The atmosphere in the dining-room, the attitudes towards school lunches and the dining-room of school staff, parents and politicians, acoustics, environment, adult participation and stress, may have a greater impact on pupils' eating habits and attitudes to food than the meal itself. The data collected in the study was in the report therefore not only related to the menu, but also to the above-mentioned, and other, factors.

Even though financial estimations were made, and were important to make, the emphasis was that there is no money to be saved, but that money could be spent in a more efficient way by being relocated from scrap waste and surplus to food eaten.

It became evident that the average amount of food taken by all age groups, all meals, (in kilograms) per person, was not sufficient, compared to the recommendations made by the nutritionist for students aged 10-13. The amount of scrap waste per person increased with the age of the students, from 5% to 18%. There was a daily surplus ordered from the central kitchen of approximately

20%. The crowded dining rooms had the most scrap waste, 17-18% of taken food. A financial estimation of scrap waste per person in the different age groups (ranging from 0.19kr to 1.60kr.) was made. Attendance decreased with the age of the students, from 95% to 60%. Only two dining-rooms served salads in accordance with the national nutritional guidelines. Four out of six school cafeterias were open during the lunch period.

A political decision was taken to promote the implementation of national guidelines for school lunches, which include, amongst many things, offering a second main course, as well as a variety of salads and side courses, lunch to be served after 11 o'clock and at the same time every day for classes.

It is suggested that it will be important to build on the common goal, interest and responsibility of all participants (kitchen and dining-room staff, school administrators, politicians, parents, students, personnel department, real estate department) in the system as opposed to them being audited and evaluated individually. It is also recommended that there is a need to link research findings from other studies to the local hard data, such as the comparison between how much should be eaten and how much was eaten. This link could also be extended to other features such as what should be served and what was served, safety regulations and number of people in dining-room. There is a clear need to make financial estimations of waste and surplus, thereby creating a strong incentive for change.

I wish to bring you my thoughts in drawing our forum to a conclusion.

Clearly the school is a good starting point for nutrition action but **coherence** is important. By coherence I mean the connections to related areas, which impact on health eating such as the family, wider society and external influences or the supply of food in supermarkets.

We need to listen to **the voice of young people** as exemplified by the Young Minds project. In their eyes the following issues are important in the choices young people make about food:

- pricing policy – make the healthy choices easier;

- managing the eating environment – features such as queues are important;

- creating an image – healthy food may not be cool;

- use innovative techniques such as ICT (information/communication technology);

- nutrition is a technical term we need to recognise the social function of food;

Young people (and all people) perceive food in terms of healthiness - but also in terms of satisfying hunger, enjoyment, style and brand, and the many social functions of eating.

We need to recognise **the different social, cultural and historical factors** that have produced different approaches to supply food in schools across Europe.

In some countries, for example Finland, Sweden, Scotland, England, Wales, France and Slovenia, we have policy laid down at a national level. In other countries such as Norway, Denmark, the Netherlands, Germany and Austria, there is a local or regional flexibility in terms of food provision.

It could be argued that policy is important at all levels – the classroom, school, community and at national level.

There are implications from this seminar **for further research and development work.** These can be summarised as follows:

- papers, posters and discussions will be published in a report.

- A task force will discuss which recommendations and practical guidelines are required as a result of the forum

- Researchers will meet after this forum to discuss research challenges.

We need to build better links with the **food industry**. For example, encouraging:

- healthy snack production;
- organic, vegetarian and ethnic varieties;
- corporate nutritional responsibility;
- partnerships;
- working with food processors as well as contractors.

Specific practical ideas, which have been suggested at the forum:

- benchmarking of school meal systems;
- ratio divided vending machines;
- fizzy drink-free days;
- the need to learn from fast food marketing ;
- local food events as a stimulus for change.

Issues to be recognised:

- the students are consumers;
- changing role of parents and families;
- the overloaded curriculum;
- perception of a health/'joie de vivre' tension

At the **international** level, we need to draw together our learning and experience and co-operate on research. There will be a follow-up meeting at the end of the seminar to consider international research proposals to the European Commission.

As I stated earlier, we need to build on our successes such as the growth of fruit and vegetable promotions and develop our networks of communication to which this forum has made a contribution. We also need to consider sharing our education programmes and develop future recommendations and guidelines as a result of this forum.

As the rapporteur of the forum I have had the task of editing the contributions and integrating the events at the forum into this report.

I should make it clear that all of the papers have been edited by me to some extent because of the constraints of space and the need to have a degree of consistency in the style and tone of the report. In some cases fuller versions of the papers are to be found in the Proceedings of the forum published by the Council of Europe on its website (Appendix 3). In other cases the version in this report is more substantial, either because the original in the provisional proceedings was an abstract or because I have added additional material from the presentation actually given at the event. This was quite a complex task and it was not possible in the time available to give edited text back to all the authors, which I trust will be understood by them. If any reader wishes further information on any of the papers the authors may be contacted directly (participants' email addresses Appendix 1).

There was a strong feeling at the seminar that we are at a crossroads in relation to healthy eating. The rapid increase in obesity in young people has raised the political profile of the issue and this was reflected in the media interest in the forum. At the international level the WHO and the Council of Europe have demonstrated commitment. As one of the participants said in their evaluation forum "Thanks for organising this event!"

Throughout Europe there is evidence of a huge range of research and development projects relating to food in schools and in policy developments in several countries at the national level. There are significant cultural differences which emerged at the forum which were not fully discussed. For example, the promotion of organic food is viewed by many delegates as a positive trend. This seemed to be a high priority for some delegates but it is perceived as a more peripheral issue by the mainstream scientific community in other countries. Similarly the difference of views expressed on whether a lunchbox or packed lunch was adequate compared to a hot meal was touched on but not teased out.

However, putting aside these differences there was broad consensus on many of the major issues such as the need to effectively promote fruit and vegetables or the need to take a whole-school approach to influence what young people, and the whole school community, are eating.

The scope of the issues that were discussed at the event were encompassed by the diverse themes of the posters. There were papers on the themes of policy, partnership, education, research, traditions and the environment. There was also recognition at the forum that in policy terms the promotion of healthy eating has to involve schools but that this is only part of a solution, which has to be inter-sectoral.

The following points emerged as key issues.

- A whole school or health promoting school approach should be used. Research makes clear the limitations of a curriculum-only approach and the benefits of a whole school approach.

- Policy development needs to engage and involve young people and take account of the realities of their lives inside and outside school.

- We need to offer young people choices in relation to food. We can develop policies and strategies that facilitate the healthy choices. Good examples of this were given at the forum.

- Given the many important roles food plays in our lives, we should move from talking about nutrition education to focussing on the promotion of healthy eating.

- Healthy eating policies need to consider environmental issues in relation to food production. In a Europe and biosphere of diminishing natural resources this issue will become much more important in the future.

- The role of the training of teachers and food providers was demonstrated as central to success in several initiatives. We need to consider innovative ways of making training available and accessible to key partners, which acknowledges the limited time available in pre-service training.

- The evidence is emerging that partnership work is the way ahead. However it is complex and requires a great investment in time. We need to understand the factors, which may promote or inhibit partnerships.

- We need to build on the good examples of partnerships with parents, young people, teachers, food producers and cross-sectoral government agencies.

- There is a need to review the existing research evidence on effectiveness. In my view we already know which methodologies are most likely to be effective in promoting healthy eating, but we need to make this case concisely for politicians and policy makers.

- The methodologies that are effective for promoting healthy eating will normally be shared with other topic-related areas such as physical activity and smoking prevention. This is a reminder that we need to take a holistic approach to aspects of our policy development.

- Healthy food provision at school is about human ecology as well as nutrition in a narrower sense. Policy development therefore has to take account of the young person's interaction with the school physical environment and social environment. This would include the students' views on queuing, seating and music in the dining-room and the myriad of factors that influence healthy choices at school.

- Although reducing obesity is an important goal in food provision at school, we must ensure that no young person is hungry or undernourished at school.

The development of a formal resolution on food provision in schools should be considered by the Council of Europe. Such a resolution can be supportive of work both at national and local level and a powerful tool to persuade policy makers to act. This forum has provided a rich source of ideas that will be the basis of such a resolution.

If we are to take the best route from the crossroads at which we currently stand, we need policies that are based on existing good practice. In this way we can find an effective route to health promotion. There are probably no shortcuts to success as effective partnerships take time to build, but the forum has made a significant contribution and the Council of Europe should be able to take us forward to the next stage.

Task force members

Dr Bent Egberg Mikkelsen (chairman), Danish Veterinary and Food Administration

Dr Lars Ovesen (chairman until June 2003), Danish Veterinary and Food Administration

Dr Anne Marie Beck (until June 2003), Danish Veterinary and Food Administration

Mr Ian Young (rapporteur), NHS Health Scotland

Mrs Jeltje Snel, Netherlands Nutrition Centre

Mme Cristine Deliens, asbl Coordination Education et Santé, Belgium

Mrs Vivian Barnekow Rasmussen, WHO, Regional Office for Europe

Ad Hoc group members

Mrs Anniken Aarum, Directorate for Health and Social Affairs, Norway

Dr Marusa Adamic, Public Health Institute of the Republic of Slovenia

Ms Vivian Barnekow Rasmussen, WHO, Regional Office for Europe

Dr Anne Marie Beck (until June 2003), Danish Veterinary and Food Administration

Mr Elling Bere, Institute for Nutrition Research, Norway

Mrs Fannie de Boer, Wageningen University and Research Centre, the Netherlands (technical expert)

Dr Michel Chauliac, Direction Générale de la Santé, France

Mme Cristine Deliens, asbl Coordination Education et Santé. Belgium

Dr Pedro Mario Fernandez Sanjuan, National Centre of Nutrition, Spain

Dr Kaija Hasunen, Ministry of Social Affairs and Health, Finland

Prof Dr Ines Heindl, University of Flensburg, Germany (technical expert)

Dr Bent Egberg Mikkelsen (chairman), Danish Veterinary and Food Administration

Mrs Ursula O'Dwyer, Department of Health and Children, Ireland

Dr Lars Ovesen (chairman until June 2003), Danish Veterinary and Food Administration

Dr Irena Simcic, Institute of Education of the Republic of Slovenia

Mrs Jeltje Snel, Netherlands Nutrition Centre

Mrs Anna Sutter, Federal Office of Public Health, Switzerland

Mme Marie-Cécile Vadeau-Ducher, Ministère de l'Emploi et de la Solidarité, France

Prof Maria Daniel Vaz de Almeida, University of Porto, Portugal

Forum

Chair

Dr. Bent Egberg MIKKELSEN, Danish Veterinary and Food Administration
Denmark, e-mail. bem@fdir.dk

General Rapporteur

Mr Ian YOUNG, NHS Health Scotland
Scotland, Great Britain, e-mail. ian.young@hebs.scot.nhs.uk

Facilitators

Mrs Jeltje H. SNEL, Netherlands Nutrition Centre
The Netherlands, e-mail. snel@voedingscentrum.nl

Mrs Vivian BARNEKOW RASMUSSEN, World Health Organization, Regional Office for Europe
Denmark, e-mail. VBR@euro.who.int

Prof. Maria Daniel VAZ DE ALMEIDA, University of Porto
Portugal, e-mail. mdvalmeida@fcna.up.pt

Mme Cristine DELIENS, asbl Coordination Education/Santé
Belgium, e-mail. c.deliens@beon.be

Speakers

Prof. Lea MAES, University of Ghent
Belgium, e-mail. lea.maes@ugent.be

Mrs Fannie DE BOER, Wageningen University Research Centre
The Netherlands, e-mail. fannie.deboer@wur.nl

Dr Prof Ines HEINDL, University of Flensburg
Germany, e-mail. iheindl@uni-flensburg.de

Ms Gillian KYNOCH, Scottish Executive Health Department
Scotland, Great Britain, e-mail. gillian.kynoch@scotland.gsi.gov.uk

Prof Dr Isabelle LOUREIRO, Escola Nacional de Salūde Pūblica
Portugal, e-mail. isalou@ensp.unl.pt

Mr Richard COUDYSER, Sodexho Education
France, e-mail. richard.coudyser@sodexho-fr.com

Mrs Anniken OWREN AARUM, Directorate for Health and Social Affairs
Norway, e-mail. aka@shdir.no

Dr Doris KUHNESS, Styria vitalis Organisation
Austria, e-mail. gesunde.volksschule@styriavitalis.at

Mr Goof BUIJS, National Institute of Health Promotion and Disease Prevention
The Netherlands, e-mail. gbuijs@nigz.nl

Mr Jean-Claude VUILLE, Department of Public Health, City of Bern
Switzerland, e-mail. jcvuille@hin.ch

Dr Irena SIMCIC, Institute of Education of the Republic of Slovenia
Slovenia, e-mail. irena.simcic@zrss.si

Ms Cirila HLASTAN-RIBIC, Ministry of Health
Slovenia, e-mail. cirila.hlastan-ribic@gov.si

Mr Bjarne BRUUN JENSEN, University of Education
Denmark, e-mail. bjbj@dpu.dk

Mme Patricia MELOTTE, Parents' association "Clair-Vivre" Pre-Primary and Primary School, Belgium, e-mail. patricia.melotte@banksys.be

Mr Christophe CONTENT, , Parents' association "Clair-Vivre" Pre-Primary and Primary School, Belgium, e-mail. Christophe.Content@inergyautomotive.com

Mr Michel CHAULIAC, Ministry of Health
France, e-mail. michel.chauliac@sante.gouv.fr

Young Minds

Mr Friso ANNEMA, Pupil, Piter Jelles Montessori School
The Netherlands

Mrs Käthe BRUUN JENSEN, Teacher
Denmark, e-mail. Kathe.Bruun.Jensen@skolekom.dk

Mr Erik ELKHUIZEN, Pupil, Piter Jelles Montessori School
The Netherlands

Mrs Catriona FERGUSON, Teacher, Plockton High School, Ross-shire
Scotland, Great Britain

Mr Donald FERGUSON, Plockton High School, Ross-shire
Scotland, Great Britain, e-mail. donald.ferguson@highland.gov.uk

Mr Lief HOLM, DPU
Denmark, e-mail. lgh@dpu.dk

Ms Sara HUNTER, Pupil, Plockton High School, Ross-shire
Scotland, Great Britain

Ms Kaija JUMPPANEN ANDERSEN, Pupil, Målør, Municipality school
Denmark

Mr Jens H. LUND, Danish University of Education
Denmark, e-mail. Jens.Lund3@skolekom.dk

Ms Tara McARDLE, Pupil, Plockton High School, Ross-shire
Scotland, Great Britain

Mr Pyt Jon SIKKEMA, Teacher, Piter Jelles, Monteressori school
The Netherlands, e-mail. a.hekkema@wanadoo.nl

Mr Kasper WINSLØV THOMSEN, Pupil, Målør, Municipality school
Denmark

Countries

Austria

Mrs Doris DREIER, Styria vitalis Organisation

Belgium

Mrs Claire BERTHET, asbl Coordination Education et Santé
E-mail. midis.ecole@beon.be

Mr Albert D'ADESKY, Ministère Fédéral de la Santé Publique
E-mail. albert.dadesky@health.fgov.be

Mme Stéphanie HATERTE, Euralisa asbl
E-mail. euralisa@skynet.be

Ms Renate HOCHWIESER, ENSA - European Natural Soyfoods
E-mail. secretariat@ensa.be

Ms Charlotte LONFILS, Ecole de Santé Publique, Université libre de Bruxelles
E-mail. charlotte.lonfils@ulb.ac.be

Ms Mieke MIEVIS, Ministerie van de Vlaamse Gemeenschap
E-mail. mieke.mievis@wvc.vlaanderen.be

Mr Guy VALKENBORG, Ministère Fédéral de la Santé Publique
E-mail. guyvalkenborg@eas.be

Bulgaria

Mrs Donka BAYKOVA, National Centre of Hygiene, Medical Ecology and Nutrition
E-mail. d.baikova@nchmer.government.bg

Dr Nelia MIKUSHINSKA, Ministry of Health
E-mail. nmikushinska@mh.government.bg

Mlle Denitsa PANCHEVA, Ministry of Youth and Sports
E-mail. denipanch@youthsport.bg

Prof. Stefka PETROVA, national centre of hygiene
E-mail. s.petrova@nchmen.government.bg

Denmark

Mrs Kirsten BLICHER FRIIS, Det Gode Maltid
E-mail. kirstenbf@roskildekom.dk

Mrs Astrid DAHL, Technical University of Denmark
E-mail. ad@ipl.dtu.dk

Mrs Karen ERIKSEN, Danish Veterinary and Food Administration
E-mail. Keri@fdir.dk

Ms Maria HAUKROGH, Danish Veterinary and Food Administration
E-mail. MHAU@FDIR.DK

Mrs Gitte HOLM, Øddannelelses og Ungdomsforvaltningen
E-mail. Gitteholm@uuf.kk.dk

Dr Ster Heine KRISTENSEN, Technical University of Denmark
E-mail. nhk@ipl.dtu.dk

Mrs Lene KROMANN-LARSEN, The Danish Heart Foundation
E-mail. lklarsen@hjerteforeningen.dk

Mr Jan MICHELSEN, UUF
E-mail. jmi@uuf.kk.dk

Mrs Nina NIELSEN, Ministry of Education
E-mail. ninie1@uvm.dk

Ms Mine SYLOW, Danish Veterinary and Food Administration
E-mail. mxsp@fdir.dk

Mrs Tove VESTERGAARD, Danish Veterinary and Food Administration
E-mail. tvl@fdir.dk

Finland

Dr Kaija HARTIALA, Deputy Mayor, City of Turku
E-mail. kaija.hartiala@turku.fi

Dr Kaija HASUNEN, Ministry of Social Affairs and Health
E-mail. kaija.hasunen@stm.vn.fi

Mrs Ulla Marja URHO, Dairy Nutrition Council
E-mail. ulla-marja.urho@etl.fi

France

Mme Agnès BONIFAY, Compass Group
E-mail. agnès.bonifay@compass-group.fr

Mr Bernard CHARDON, Sodexho
E-mail. ChardonJB@aol.com

Mr Michel CLEVENOT, Rectorat de Strasbourg
E-mail. michel.clevenot@ac-strasbourg.fr

Mme Brigitte COUDRAY, CERIN
E-mail. bcoudray@cerin.org

Mme Corinne DELAMAIRE, INPES
E-mail. corinne.delamaire@inpes.sante.fr

Mme Cécile DE VALLOIS, CERIN
E-mail. ceciledevallois@club-internet.fr

Mr Jean-Pierre FAVREAU, Restaurants Scolaires Ville La Rochelle
E-mail. FAVREAU@ville-larochelle.fr

Mme Géraldine GEFFROY, Compass Group France
E-mail. geraldine.geffroy@compass-group.fr

Mme Virginie GRANDJEAN, Centre d'Information des Viandes
E-mail. v.grandjean@civ-viande.org

Mme Andrée HASSELMANN, Ville de Strasbourg, Service Education
E-mail. ahasselmann@cus-strasbourg.net

Mr Christophe HEBERT, Association Nationale des Directeurs de la Restauration
Municipale, E-mail. hebertch@wanadoo.fr

Dr Francine HIRTZ, Inspection Académique des Yvelines
E-mail. francine.hirtz@ac-versailles.fr

Dr Jeanne KOCHANOWSKI, Service Médical du Rectorat de l'Académie de
Strasbourg, E-mail. jeanne.kochanowski@ac-strasbourg.fr

Dr Dominique LALANNE, Inspection Académique, Service Médical
E-mail. catherine.gavend@ac-lyon.fr

Dr Nathalie LESPLINGARD, Comité Régional d'Education pour la Santé de Basse-
Normandie, E-mail. cresbn14@hotmail.com

Mlle Valérie MARCHAL, Association Départementale d'Education Sanitaire et
Sociale de Savoie, E-mail. vmarchal@sante-savoie.org

Mme Christiane MASLANKA, APASP (Association pour l'achat dans les services
publics), E-mail. apasp@apasp.com

Mr Daniel MASLANKA, Rectorat de l'Académie de Lille
E-mail. daniel.maslanka@uc-lille.fr

Dr Sophie TREPPOZ, A.F.P.A. (Association française de Pédiatrie), and A.P.O.P.
(Association pour la Prise en charge et la Prévention de l'Obésité en Pédiatrie)
E-mail. softreppoz@aol.com

Mr Michel VUILLEROD, Groupe Danone
E-mail. mvuiller@groupe.danone.com

Mme Florence WARENGHEM, Services de Promotion de la Santé et de l'Action
Sociale en Faveur des Elèves, E-mail. Ce.la73-SMS@ac-grenoble.fr

Germany

Ms Michaela BAHR, University of Applied Sciences
E-mail. Michaela.Baehr@rzbd.haw-hamburg.de

Prof. Dr. Dieter BEGER, Fachhochschule für Öffentliche Verwaltung and Member of the Board of Ökomarkt, Ökomarkt Verbraucher und Agrarberatung e.V.
E-mail. Beger@oekomarkt-hamburg.de

Ms Angela BORCHERT, HAW Hamburg
E-mail. angela.borchert@rzbd.haw-hamburg.de

Prof. Dr. Helmut LABERENZ, University of Applied Sciences
E-mail. Helmut.Laberenz@rzbd.haw-hamburg.de

Ms Costanza MÜLLER, Ökomarkt Verbraucher und Agrarberatung e.V.
E-mail. Mueller@oekomarkt-hamburg.de

Prof. Olaf-W NAATZ, University of Applied Sciences
E-mail. Olaf.W.Naatz@rzbd.haw-hamburg.de

Mrs Angela M. RUSACK, apetito bv
E-mail. Angela.Rusack@apetito.de

Dr Carola STRASSNER, Organic Foodservice Consultancy
E-mail. carola.strassner@oegs.de

Ms Christiane THEOPHILE, University of Applied Sciences
E-mail. Christiane.Theophile@rzbd.haw-hamburg.de

Hungary

Prof Maria BARNA, Hungarian Society of Nutrition
E-mail. drbarnam@hotmail.com

Prof Imre RODLER, Hungarian Society of Nutrition
E-mail. h8649rod@ella.hu

Mr Gabor ZAJKAS, NTL Institute of Food Hygiene and Nutrition
E-mail. h11447zaj@ella.hu

Ireland

Mrs Ursula O'DWYER, Department of Health and Children
E-mail. ursula_o'dwyer@health.irlgov.ie

Italy

Dr Ersilia TROIANO, Italian Society of Human Nutrition (SINU)
E-mail. ersilia_troiano@libero.it

Latvia

Mr Uldis ARMANIS, Latvian Food Centre
E-mail. uldis.armanis@lpc.gov.lv

Luxembourg

Mr Jeff HEYART, Professeur de Biologie
E-mail. jeff.heyart@education.lu

Mrs Liz MERSCH, Centre thermal et de santé
E-mail. l.mersch@mondorf.lu

Dr Margot MULLER, Division de la Médecine Scolaire
E-mail. margot.muller@ms.etat.lu

Mme Sylvie PAQUET, Direction de la Santé
E-mail. sylvie.paquet@ms.etat.lu

Norway

Mrs Aase Marie RUSAANES, Ministry of Agriculture
E-mail. ase-marie.rusaanes@ld.dep.no

Ms Bodil BLAKER, Ministry of Health
E-mail. bob@hd.dep.no

Mrs Grete HAUG, National Board of Education
E-mail. grete.haug@ls.no

Poland

Mrs Maria SOKOLOWSKA, Methodical Centre psycho-pedagogical assistance
E-mail. pez@CMPPP.EDU.PL

Portugal

Mrs Bela FRANCHINI, Faculty of Nutrition and Food Sciences, Oporto University
E-mail belafranchini@fcna.up.pt

Mrs Madalena B. PEREIRA, Ministère de l'Education
E-mail. madapereira@mail.telepac.pt

Dr Teresa SOARES DA SILVA, Oporto Educational Centre
E-mail. mtssilva@oninet.pt

Mrs Ester Maria VINHA NOVA, Gabinete Nutricao - Sub-Regiao de Saude Viseu
E-mail. gabnutri@srsviseu.min-saude.pt

Republic of Moldova

Mr Guttul AUREL, National Centre of Preventive Medicine
E-mail. aguttul@mednet.md

Spain

Dr Pedro Mario FERNÁNDEZ SAN JUAN, Centro Nacional de Alimentación AESA
E-mail. pmariof@isciii.es

Dr Carmen PEREZ RODRIGO, Subarea Municipal de Salud Publica
E-mail. bisaludpublica@wanadoo.es

Sweden

Ms Mette KJÖRSTAD, Public Health Administrator, Tyresö Municipality
E-mail. mette.kjorstad@tyreso.se

Switzerland

Mrs Anna SUTTER, Federal Office of Public Health
E-mail. anna.sutter@bag.admin.ch

The Netherlands

Mrs Ria VAN DER MAES, Unilever R & D Vlaardingen
E-mail. Ria-van-der.Maas@unilever.com

Mrs Marja SLAGMOOLEN-GYZE, Holland Produce Promotion
E-mail. m.slagmoolen@agfpn.nl

Mr Bauke HOUTSMA, Groenhorst College
E-mail. b.houtsma@planet.nl

Mr Ferdy NAAFS, Dutch Association of Public Authority Education (VOO)
E-mail. FNAAFS@VOO.nl

Ms Beeltje LIEFERS, FMO
E-mail. b.liefers@fmobv.nl

United Kingdom

Mr Tony APICELLA, Out of School Hours Learning, England
E-mail. tony.apicella@continyou.org.uk

Mrs Sue BOWKER, Health Promotion Division Welsh Assembly Government, Wales, E-mail. Sue.bowker@wales.gsi.gov.uk

Mrs Courtney COOKE, NHS Health Scotland, Scotland
E-mail. courtney.cooke@hebs.scot.nhs.uk

Mrs Francesca FANUCCI, Ergo Communications, England
E-mail fanuccif@ergo-c.com

Mrs Sara FORD, Department for Education and Skills, England
E-mail sara.ford@dfes.gsi.gov.uk

Mr Rob HANCOCK, Kent County Council, England
E-mail rob.hancock@kent.gov.uk

Mr Mark KARACZUN, North Norfolk Primary Care Trust, England
E-mail. Mark.Karaczun@norfolk.nhs.uk

Mrs Alison MACKWAY, 5-a-Day Co-ordinator, England
E-mail. Alison.Mackway@norfolk.nhs.uk

Mrs Patricia McCusker, Department of Education for Northern Ireland, N. Ireland
E-mail mccuskerpatricia@hotmail.com

Dr Lynne McMULLAN, Department of Education for Northern Ireland, N. Ireland
E-mail lynne.mcmullan@deni.gov.uk

Mrs Catherine PICKETT, Welsh Assembly Government, Wales
E-mail Catherine.pickett@wales.gsi.gov.uk

Dr Jennifer WOOLFE, Food Standards Agency, England
E-mail jenny.woolfe@foodstandards.gsi.gov.uk

Ms Rachel THOM, Department of Health, England
E-mail rachel.thom@doh.gsi.gov.uk

Observers

Parliamentary Assembly of the Council of Europe

Mr Mike HANCOCK (apologized/excusé), United Kingdom Parliament
E-mail hancockm@parliament.uk

World Health Organization

Dr Aileen ROBERTSON, Regional Office for Europe, Denmark
E-mail aro@who.dk

European Commission

Mr Wilfried KAMPHAUSEN, Direction Générale Santé et Protection et
des consommateurs, Luxembourg
E-mail Wilfried.Kamphausen@cec.eu.int

Grouping "Education Culture" NGO

Mr Alain MOUCHOUX, Regroupement d'ONG "Education et Culture", France
E-mail Secretariat@csee-etuce.org

Press

Mme Sonia WOLF, Agence France Presse
E-mail sonia.wolf@afp.com

Mr Denis DURAND DE BOUSINGEN, Le Quotidien du Médecin
E-mail bousingen@web.de

Mr Joel WOLCHOVER, Catchline News Agency
E-mail joel@catchlinenews.co.uk

Secretariat

DG III – Social Cohesion
Department of Health and of the Partial Agreement in the Social and Public Health Field

Fax number: +33 (0)3 88 41 27 32
Website: www.coe.int/soc-sp

Dr Peter BAUM, Head of Division
E-mail. peter.baum@coe.int

Mr Laurent LINTERMANS, Administrative Officer
E-mail. laurent.lintermans@coe.int

Ms Sheila BOULAJOUN, Principal Administrative Assistant
E-mail. sheila.boulajoun@coe.int

Ms Audrey MALAISE, Assistant
E-mail. audrey.malaise@coe.int

Ms Jane-Lindsay CHESTNUTT, Assistant

Health Division

Web site: www.coe.int/T/E/Social_Cohesion/Health/
Fax number: + 33 (03) 88 41 27 26

Mr. Karl-Friedrich BOPP, Head of Division
E-mail. karl-friedrich.bopp@coe.int

Interpreters

Mme Josette YOESLE-BLANC

Mme Sylvie BOUX

Mme Monique PALMIER

1. **Healthy eating at school – an integrated nutrition education project in a Portuguese junior school**; Teresa Soares da Silva, Maria Daniel Vaz de Almeida, and Maria do Céu Taveira; Portugal.
   E-mail. mtssilva@oninet.pt

2. **The impact of a nutrition education program**; E. Alves de Almeida MDV; Portugal.
   E-mail. mdvalmeida@fcna.up.pt

3. **Interactive CD-Rom: discover healthy eating**; B. Francini, P. Graça, L. Sá, P. Queiroz, L. Rodrigues, and M. D. Vaz de Almeida; Portugal.
   E-mail. belafranchini@fcna.up.pt

4. **Measures to improve nutrition in schools in Wales**; S. Bowker, and C. Pickett; United Kingdom.
   E-mail. Sue.Bowker@wales.gsi.gov.uk

5. **Developing sustainable strategies to promote healthy eating across the school day in England**; R. L. Thom; United Kingdom.
   E-mail. Rachel.thom@doh.gsi.gov.uk

6. **Research aimed at promoting healthier eating in children**; J. A. Woolfe; United Kingdom.
   E-mail. jenny.woolfe@foodstandards.gsi.gov.uk

7. **A training resource – growing through adolescence: a health promoting school approach to healthy eating**; Monica Merson, Courtney Cooke, Rachael Roberts, Ian Young, Candace Currie, and Jo Inchley; United Kingdom.
   E-mail. ian.young@hebs.scot.nhs.uk

8. **Food can only provide energy when eaten; intake of school lunches;** Mette Kjörstad; Sweden.
   E-mail. mette.kjorstad@tyreso.se

9. **"Dime come comes": a joint initiative between the catering sector and public health nutrition**; J. Aranceta, C. Perez-Rodrigo, L. I. Serra-Majem, and A. Delgado; Spain.
   E-mail. bisaludpublica@wanadoo.es

10. **Monitoring program of school meals in the municipality of Bilbao**, J. Aranceta, C. Perez-Rodrigo, J. Santolaya, J. Gondra, and Bilbao School Health Group; Spain.
    E-mail. bisaludpublica@wanadoo.es

11. **Primary prevention of child obesity at infant and primary school**; Dr Nathalie Lesplinglard, and Dr Jean-Luc Vert; France.
    E-mail. cresbn14@hotmail.com

12. **Finnish school meals of 7th – 9th grade pupils**; Ulla-Marja Urho; Finland.
    E-mail. ulla-marja.urho@etl.fi

13. **Current problems in nutrition of Bulgarian schoolchildren**; S. Petrova, D. Baykova, and N. Mikushinska; Bulgaria.
    E-mail. S.Petrova@nchmen.government.bg

14. **Preliminary qualitative study of use of information by those directly involved in nutrition education projects for young people**; C. Lonfils, T. Nguyen, and D. Piette; Belgium.
    E-mail. charlotte.lonfils@ulb.ac.be

15. **Improving lunchtime at schools: building change at local level, taking account all points of view**; C. Deliens, and C. Berthet; Belgium.
    E-mail. c.deliens@beon.be

16. **"Diet in a nutshell – a taste for life" development of healthy eating at school – a regional approach**; Maria Haukrogh; Denmark.
    E-mail. MHAU@FDIR.DK

17. **Healthy and organic school food for 30,000 schoolchildren in Copenhagen**; Gitte Holm, and Jan Michelsen; Denmark.
    E-mail. Gitteholm@uuf.kk.dk

18. **Partnership between authorities and NGOs in developing healthy eating at school – the Danish experience**; B. E. Mikkelsen, K. Skovsby, and L. M. Christensen; Denmark.
    E-mail. bem@fdir.dk

19. **'The good meal': improving public meals and public food provision**; Kirsten Blicher Friis; Denmark.
    E-mail. kirstenbf@roskildekom.dk

20. **A qualitative study of barriers to healthy food for children in Danish day-care centres and schools**; L. M. Christensen, B. E. Mikkelsen, and K. Skovsby; Denmark.
    E-mail. bem@fdir.dk

21. **Promoting good school cafeterias in secondary schools through nutrition action teams**; Jeltje Snel, and Anne Maaike Reitzema; the Netherlands.
    E-mail. snel@voedingscentrum.nl

22. **National fruit and vegetable project for primary schools in the Netherlands**; M. Slagmoolen, M. Luchinger, and E. van der Ham; the Netherlands.
    E-mail. m.slagmoolen@agfpn.nl

23. **Schoolbeat: a collaborative approach to co-ordinated school health promotion in the Netherlands**; Mariken Leurs, Maria Jansen, Goof Buijs, and Herman Schaalma; the Netherlands.
    E-mail. M_Leurs@zzl-ggd.nl

24. **Pilot warm meals in primary schools during lunchtime**; F. Naafs; the Netherlands.
    E-mail. FNAAFS@VOO.nl

25. **Appropriate terms of reference for public invitations to tender for school catering**; C. Strassner, A. Erhart, and R. Roehl; Germany
    E-mail. carola.strassner@oegs.de

26. **Effect of a fruit and vegetable subscription in Danish schools**; K. Eriksen, J. Haraldsdóttir, R. Pederson, H. Vig Flyger; Denmark

APPENDIX 3: SOME USEFUL WEBSITES

The following websites were either referred to in presentations and in discussion sessions or were submitted to the rapporteur as useful sites by participants at the forum. The list is obviously not comprehensive and the inclusion of an address does not imply any formal endorsement by the Council of Europe. However many of them will prove useful to readers of this report.

www.coe.int/soc-sp

www.euro.who.int/nutrition

www.who.int/gb/EB_WHA/PDF/EB113/eeb11344.al.pdf
(the above is the draft global strategy on diet, physical activity and health)

www.euro.who.int/HFADB

www.wbln.0018.worldbank.org

www.euro.dk/ENHPS

www.europa.eu.int

www.hbsc.org

www.unicef.org

www.fao.org

www.young-minds.net

www.eufic.org

www.daisy.at

www.styriavitalis.at

www.afsca.be

www.sante.cfwb.be

www.ulb.ac.be/esp/promes

www.nubel.com

www.motives.be

www.atablecartable.be

www.vig.be

www.vlam.be

www.dge.de

www.gesundeschule.ch

www.bern.ch

www.altomkost.dk

hhtp://perso.wanadoo.fr/andrm

www.sante.gouv.fr

www.inpes.santé.fr

www.pipsa.org

www.centre-evian.com

www.danoneinstitute.org/home/index.php

www.danonevitapole.com/extranet/vitapole/portail.nsf

www.egmondconference.nl

www.nigz.nl

www.schoolslag.nl

www.voedingscentrum.nl

www.schoolgruiten.nl

www.ios-ensac.nl

www.wiredforhealth.gov.uk

www.food.gov.uk

www.nutrition.org.uk

www.doh.gov.uk/fiveaday

www.eafl.org.uk

www.fiveadaynorfolk.org

www.sustain-web.org

www.foodforlifeuk.org

www.grab5.com

www.hda-online.org.uk

www.continyou.org.uk

www.breakfast-club.co.uk

www.ifr.ac.uk/public/foodinfosheets/diet_and_cancer.html

www.pcrm.org

www.eco-schools.org.uk

www.face-online.org.uk

www.countrysidefoundation.org.uk

www.teachernet.gov.uk/growingschools

www.healtheschool.org.uk

www.healtheswales.org.uk

www.gflscotland.org.uk

www.scotland.gov.uk/Library5/education/hfs-00.asp
(school meals report, Hungry for Success)

www.healthyliving.gov.uk

www.nhshs.org

www.abdn.ac.uk/acero

Sales agents for publications of the Council of Europe
Agents de vente des publications du Conseil de l'Europe

AUSTRALIA/AUSTRALIE
Hunter Publications, 58A, Gipps Street
AUS-3066 COLLINGWOOD, Victoria
Tel.: (61) 3 9417 5361
Fax: (61) 3 9419 7154
E-mail: Sales@hunter-pubs.com.au
http://www.hunter-pubs.com.au

BELGIUM/BELGIQUE
La Librairie européenne SA
50, avenue A. Jonnart
B-1200 BRUXELLES 20
Tel.: (32) 2 734 0281
Fax: (32) 2 735 0860
E-mail: info@libeurop.be
http://www.libeurop.be

Jean de Lannoy
202, avenue du Roi
B-1190 BRUXELLES
Tel.: (32) 2 538 4308
Fax: (32) 2 538 0841
E-mail: jean.de.lannoy@euronet.be
http://www.jean-de-lannoy.be

CANADA
Renouf Publishing Company Limited
5369 Chemin Canotek Road
CDN-OTTAWA, Ontario, K1J 9J3
Tel.: (1) 613 745 2665
Fax: (1) 613 745 7660
E-mail: order.dept@renoufbooks.com
http://www.renoufbooks.com

CZECH REPUBLIC/
RÉPUBLIQUE TCHÈQUE
Suweco Cz Dovoz Tisku Praha
Ceskomoravska 21
CZ-18021 PRAHA 9
Tel.: (420) 2 660 35 364
Fax: (420) 2 683 30 42
E-mail: import@suweco.cz

DENMARK/DANEMARK
GAD Direct
Fiolstaede 31-33
DK-1171 COPENHAGEN K
Tel.: (45) 33 13 72 33
Fax: (45) 33 12 54 94
E-mail: info@gaddirect.dk

FINLAND/FINLANDE
Akateeminen Kirjakauppa
Keskuskatu 1, PO Box 218
FIN-00381 HELSINKI
Tel.: (358) 9 121 41
Fax: (358) 9 121 4450
E-mail: akatilaus@stockmann.fi
http://www.akatilaus.akateeminen.com

FRANCE
La Documentation française
(Diffusion/Vente France entière)
124, rue H. Barbusse
F-93308 Aubervilliers Cedex
Tel.: (33) 01 40 15 70 00
Fax: (33) 01 40 15 68 00
E-mail: commandes.vel@ladocfrancaise.gouv.fr
http://www.ladocfrancaise.gouv.fr

Librairie Kléber (Vente Strasbourg)
Palais de l'Europe
F-67075 Strasbourg Cedex
Fax: (33) 03 88 52 91 21
E-mail: librairie.kleber@coe.int

GERMANY/ALLEMAGNE
AUSTRIA/AUTRICHE
UNO Verlag
Am Hofgarten 10
D-53113 BONN
Tel.: (49) 2 28 94 90 20
Fax: (49) 2 28 94 90 222
E-mail: bestellung@uno-verlag.de
http://www.uno-verlag.de

GREECE/GRÈCE
Librairie Kauffmann
28, rue Stadiou
GR-ATHINAI 10564
Tel.: (30) 1 32 22 160
Fax: (30) 1 32 30 320
E-mail: ord@otenet.gr

HUNGARY/HONGRIE
Euro Info Service
Hungexpo Europa Kozpont ter 1
H-1101 BUDAPEST
Tel.: (361) 264 8270
Fax: (361) 264 8271
E-mail: euroinfo@euroinfo.hu
http://www.euroinfo.hu

ITALY/ITALIE
Libreria Commissionaria Sansoni
Via Duca di Calabria 1/1, CP 552
I-50125 FIRENZE
Tel.: (39) 556 4831
Fax: (39) 556 41257
E-mail: licosa@licosa.com
http://www.licosa.com

NETHERLANDS/PAYS-BAS
De Lindeboom Internationale Publikaties
PO Box 202, MA de Ruyterstraat 20 A
NL-7480 AE HAAKSBERGEN
Tel.: (31) 53 574 0004
Fax: (31) 53 572 9296
E-mail: books@delindeboom.com
http://home-1-worldonline.nl/~lindeboo/

NORWAY/NORVÈGE
Akademika, A/S Universitetsbokhandel
PO Box 84, Blindern
N-0314 OSLO
Tel.: (47) 22 85 30 30
Fax: (47) 23 12 24 20

POLAND/POLOGNE
Głowna Księgarnia Naukowa
im. B. Prusa
Krakowskie Przedmiescie 7
PL-00-068 WARSZAWA
Tel.: (48) 29 22 66
Fax: (48) 22 26 64 49
E-mail: inter@internews.com.pl
http://www.internews.com.pl

PORTUGAL
Livraria Portugal
Rua do Carmo, 70
P-1200 LISBOA
Tel.: (351) 13 47 49 82
Fax: (351) 13 47 02 64
E-mail: liv.portugal@mail.telepac.pt

SPAIN/ESPAGNE
Mundi-Prensa Libros SA
Castelló 37
E-28001 MADRID
Tel.: (34) 914 36 37 00
Fax: (34) 915 75 39 98
E-mail: libreria@mundiprensa.es
http://www.mundiprensa.com

SWITZERLAND/SUISSE
Adeco – Van Diermen
Chemin du Lacuez 41
CH-1807 BLONAY
Tel.: (41) 21 943 26 73
Fax: (41) 21 943 36 05
E-mail: info@adeco.org

UNITED KINGDOM/ROYAUME-UNI
TSO (formerly HMSO)
51 Nine Elms Lane
GB-LONDON SW8 5DR
Tel.: (44) 207 873 8372
Fax: (44) 207 873 8200
E-mail: customer.services@theso.co.uk
http://www.the-stationery-office.co.uk
http://www.itsofficial.net

UNITED STATES and CANADA/
ÉTATS-UNIS et CANADA
Manhattan Publishing Company
2036 Albany Post Road
CROTON-ON-HUDSON,
NY 10520, USA
Tel.: (1) 914 271 5194
Fax: (1) 914 271 5856
E-mail: Info@manhattanpublishing.com
http://www.manhattanpublishing.com

Council of Europe Publishing/Editions du Conseil de l'Europe
F-67075 Strasbourg Cedex
Tel.: (33) 03 88 41 25 81 – Fax: (33) 03 88 41 39 10 – E-mail: publishing@coe.int – Website: http://book.coe.int